NATIONAL
CANCER
CONTROL
PROGRAMMES

POLICIES AND MANAGERIAL GUIDELINES

WORLD HEALTH ORGANIZATION

GENEVA

WHO Library Cataloguing-in-Publication Data

National cancer control programmes : policies and managerial guidelines. – 2nd ed.

1. Neoplasms – prevention and control   2. National health programs – organization and administration
3. Health policy 4. Guidelines

(ISBN 92 4 154557 7)   (NLM classification: QZ 200)

The World Health Organization welcomes requests for permission to reproduce or translate its publications, in part or in full. Applications and enquiries should be addressed to the Office of Publications, World Health Organization, Geneva, Switzerland, which will be glad to provide the latest information on any changes made to the text, plans for new editions, and reprints and translations already available.

Editing, layout and design by Health & Development Networks (HDN) · *http://www.hdnet.org*
Printed in Italy.
Cover design by Marilyn Langfeld.

TABLE OF CONTENTS

ACKNOWLEDGEMENTS

The second edition of this monograph has been produced by the Cancer Control Programme of the Department of Management of Noncommunicable Diseases which forms part of the cluster dealing with Noncommunicable Diseases and Mental Health at WHO headquarters, Geneva. It was developed following a meeting on national cancer control programmes in developing countries, held in Geneva in December 2000. Participants in this meeting, and two earlier meetings to discuss national cancer control programmes are listed at the end of this report.

Editorial guidance for both editions has been provided by Anthony Miller. Kenneth Stanley provided editorial assistance for the second edition.

A number of people, who were invited to contribute after the December 2000 meeting, reviewed specific sections and made valuable contributions. These include: David Hunter, Harvard School of Public Health; David Joranson, WHO Collaborating Center for Policy & Communications in Cancer Care; Jacob Kligerman, Brazilian National Cancer Institute; Stener Kvinnsland, International Union Against Cancer; C. Victor Levin, International Atomic Energy Agency; Neil MacDonald, Centre for Bioethics at the Clinical Research Institute of Montreal; Charles Olweny, St Boniface General Hospital; Max Parkin and R.Sankaranarayanan, International Agency for Research on Cancer; Inés Salas, University of Santiago; and, from WHO, Rafael Bengoa, Ruth Bonita, Vera Da Costa e Silva, Maximilien De Courten, JoAnne Epping-Jordan, Silvana Luciani, Nejma Macklai, Maristela Monteiro, Desmond O´Byrne, Sonia Pagliusi Uhe, Pirjo Pietinen, Pekka Puska, Eva Rehfuess, Sylvia Robles, Benedetto Saraceno, Derek Yach, Tokuo Yoshida, and Mohamed Maged Younes.

The team members from the Programme on Cancer Control who worked on this edition were Amanda Marlin, Cecilia Sepúlveda and Andreas Ullrich. Secretarial work was done by Maryann Akpama. The report was edited by Angela Haden and Health & Development Networks. Layout and design by Health & Development Networks.

Executive Summary

MESSAGE FROM THE DIRECTOR-GENERAL
OF THE WORLD HEALTH ORGANIZATION

Cancer. The word still conjures up deep fears of a silent killer that creeps up on us without warning. Cancer, evoking such desperation that it has become a metaphor for grief and pain, a scourge straining our intellectual and emotional resources. The numbers are such that each of us will be touched either as a patient, a family member or a friend. There are over 20 million people living with cancer in the world today. The majority live in the developing world.

Yet, there is much that can be done in every country to prevent, cure and relieve this suffering. With the existing knowledge it is possible to prevent at least one-third of the 10 million cancer cases that occur annually throughout the world. Where sufficient resources are available, current knowledge also allows the early detection and effective treatment of a further one-third of those cases. Pain relief and palliative care can improve the quality of life of cancer patients and their families, even in very low resource settings thanks to effective, low-cost approaches.

Understanding and controlling malignant disease have very broad dimensions. It involves scientific knowledge and experience ranging from the complexities of intracellular molecular regulation to individual lifestyle choices. It also requires competent management and the best use of available resources for planning, implementing and evaluating disease control strategies. Cancer prevention and control are among the most important scientific and public health challenges of this era.

Our goal is to reduce the morbidity and mortality from cancer and improve the quality of life of cancer patients and their families, everywhere in the world where the cancer burden is high or there are rising trends of cancer risk factors. We have learned that no matter what resource constraints a country faces, a well-conceived, well-managed national cancer control programme is able to lower cancer incidence and improve the lives of people living with cancer. A comprehensive national cancer programme evaluates the various ways to control disease and implements those that are the most cost-effective and beneficial for the largest part of the population. It should promote the development of treatment guidelines, place emphasis on preventing cancers or detecting cases early so that they can be cured, and provide as much comfort as possible to patients with advanced disease.

We already know that at least one-third of all the new cases of cancer every year can be prevented. Tobacco, the single largest preventable cause of cancer in the world today, is responsible for about 30% of all cancer deaths in developed countries and a rapidly rising proportion in developing countries and in underprivileged communities. It is the only consumer product available which kills half its regular users.

In addition to strong, comprehensive tobacco control measures, dietary modification is another important approach to cancer control. Overweight and obesity are both serious risk factors for cancer. Diets high in fruits and vegetables may reduce the risk for several types of cancer, while high levels of preserved and red meat consumption are associated with increased cancer risk.

Our era has seen and continues to see great scientific advances in cancer treatment. Treatment for some cancer sites is becoming increasingly effective, yet poor availability of treatment and delays in seeking medical attention contribute to lower survival rates in many developing countries. Increasing awareness of the signs and symptoms of cancer is important to facilitate early detection of the disease. Where appropriate tests and facilities are available, screening of apparently healthy individuals can disclose cancer in early or precursor stages, where treatment may be most effective. But all too often, limited resources are used to treat patients with far-advanced disease, who really do not benefit from the treatment.

We have also learned important lessons in the field of palliative care. Millions of people around the world suffer not only from cancer, but from other chronic, life-threatening conditions in advanced stages. In these cases where prevention efforts have failed and patients and their families have little access to curative treatment, the devastation is great. These diseases affect people on all human dimensions: physical, psychological, social and spiritual. Solitude and stigma only add to physical suffering. Fortunately, there are low-cost, community approaches that can reduce this suffering and meet this urgent humanitarian need. Measures for good palliative care are essential elements in every national cancer control programme.

WHO's approach to noncommunicable disease prevention and control places emphasis on the rising impact of cancer in low-income and middle-income countries, and the disproportionate suffering it causes in poor and disadvantaged populations. Two years ago we reviewed the progress in implementing national cancer control programmes, as part of a strategy launched about a decade ago. Based on experience from Member States and our collaboration with other partners, we discussed the strengths and constraints of this strategy. While many Member States recognize the need to develop national cancer control programmes, few in the industrialized world and even fewer in developing countries have yet done so. As a result many people die from preventable cancers and suffer unnecessarily from pain and anguish at the end of their lives.

Lack of a comprehensive, systematic approach, weaknesses in organization and priority-setting, and inefficient use of resources are obstacles to effective programmes in both industrialized and developing countries. In far too many cases, primary prevention, early detection and palliative care are neglected in favor of treatment-oriented approaches, regardless of whether they are actually cost-effectiveness or whether they improve patients' quality of life. This happens because of lack of knowledge, lack of political will and lack of national capacity in policy development and programme implementation.

I believe it is the responsibility of the World Health Organization to dig deep to find the best knowledge on cancer control and to facilitate the sharing of successful country experiences among governments and other partners. As the world's leading repository of public health knowledge, we are committed to translating this knowledge into action. But we must work with others – health is a shared responsibility.

We have initiated a process for promoting and reinforcing the development of national cancer control programmes as the best known strategy to address the cancer problem worldwide. Updating and disseminating effective policies and guidelines on national cancer control programmes and providing guidance on the development of these programmes are key components of this strategy.

This document presents WHO's latest recommendations and findings. This edition will provide an updated framework for policy development and programme management that can be adapted to socioeconomic and cultural contexts in all countries. It provides the information needed to guide the development of feasible, equitable, sustainable, and effective national cancer control programmes.

I know what we are seeking to do is not easy. But the constraints and difficulties are far outweighed by the opportunities to reduce the death and suffering caused by cancer. I hope this report makes a contribution to ending the isolation and desperation of cancer patients on the one hand and strengthening national options for comprehensive cancer control on the other. I believe we can act, and we must.

Gro Harlem Brundtland
Geneva
May 2002

PREFACE FROM THE SECRETARY GENERAL OF THE INTERNATIONAL UNION AGAINST CANCER

CANCER IS AND WILL BECOME an increasingly important factor in the global burden of disease in the decades to come. The estimated number of new cases each year is expected to rise from 10 million in 2000 to 15 million by 2020. Some 60% of all these new cases will occur in the less developed parts of the world.

Improved cancer control will, to a substantial degree, relate to prevention strategies and early detection programmes, including information campaigns and population-based screening programmes. Success of the early detection programmes will rely on effective and optimal use of treatment possibilities. In spite of the explosion in knowledge of tumour biology, another decade will probably elapse before its application through new drugs and treatment principles will significantly reduce cancer mortality. The aspects of cancer control must therefore be seen within the context of a systematic and comprehensive approach, that is, the cancer control plan or strategy.

Forces in the fight against cancer include the government sector, the nongovernmental sector, the private sector and the professional organizations. Their common objective is to reduce morbidity and mortality from cancer. Each sector plays an important role within a national cancer control programme/plan/strategy, though the relative extent of that role varies depending on the situation in the country.

The nongovernmental sector is involved in cancer research, cancer registration, cancer prevention activities, treatment and care facilities, and programmes. This involvement implies either direct provision of the services or acting as funding institutions. Again, the extent of the different activities will vary from country to country. In some countries, funds for treatment come from the national government and funds for disease prevention and screening come from the state government. In other countries, nongovernmental organizations focus on the prevention and early detection of cancer. It is very important for all organizations to be aware of the complexity of cancer control, and of the role they should play in achieving the goals of the cancer control programme or strategy, through a unified effort with other sectors.

The nongovernmental sector is an important source of technical know-how, skills and resources relevant for cancer care and research. Furthermore, nongovernmental organizations provide an important ability to reach out to the professional and public communities. Community participation in cancer care is essential. This need is particularly acute in the developing countries, given the constrained resources and operational limitations of the government health care systems. Major portions of healthcare budgets in developing countries, which are largely insufficient to begin with, are dedicated to the control of communicable diseases, leaving small margins for allocation to noncommunicable disease control programmes. Nongovernmental and voluntary organizations can, therefore, play a significant role in assisting the efforts of the government health system in reducing disparities in coverage with regard to cancer care services.

In close collaboration with the World Health Organization, the International Union Against Cancer (UICC) promotes the participation of nongovernmental organizations in the development and implementation of national and regional cancer control strategies, and helps to build the capacity in these organizations in the areas of cancer prevention and early detection, particularly through educational and training programmes. By its participation in establishing a national cancer control strategy or plan, the nongovernmental sector will be able to better understand its own role in providing cancer care services, including support of cancer research. The comprehensive and systematic approach to the cancer problem, as presented in a national cancer control programme, gives all providers of cancer care and research the optimal possibility of giving the right focus and proportions to their own work.

The second edition of the WHO publication on national cancer control programmes is an important tool in promoting cancer control strategies. The different elements of a cancer plan are well described, and appropriate organizational aspects discussed. As was the case with the first edition, this publication will be of great value for the establishment and implementation of national cancer control plans.

Stener Kvinnsland
Oslo
May 2002

FOREWORD

THIS MONOGRAPH aims to provide a framework for the development of national cancer control programmes. Its underlying approach is the application of science to public health practice, providing a concise statement of what is feasible and desirable in cancer prevention and control, with the ultimate goal of reducing cancer morbidity and mortality, and improving quality of life in the targeted population. It is intended primarily for policymakers in health and related fields, but will also be of interest to health ministries and academic institutions and, more generally, to oncologists and other health professionals who need to be aware of developments in cancer control.

The first edition of this monograph was produced following the meeting of a Working Group on National Cancer Control Programmes, 25–29 November 1991, at WHO headquarters in Geneva, Switzerland. The second edition of this monograph has been produced by the Cancer Control Programme of the Department of Management of Noncommunicable Diseases, WHO, following a meeting on national cancer control programmes in developing countries, held in Geneva in December 2000. Editorial guidance for both editions has been provided by Professor Anthony B. Miller. Dr Kenneth Stanley provided editorial assistance for the second edition. We would also like to acknowledge the seminal work of Dr Jan Stjernswärd, former Chief of the WHO Cancer Unit. While it is not possible to acknowledge all contributions of the countless individuals and organizations that gave so freely of their expertise, the participants at the major WHO meetings on the theme of this monograph are listed at the end of this report.

The timeliness of this updated publication is underlined by the fact that the World Health Organization has designated noncommunicable diseases, including cancer, as a priority area. Moreover, WHO Member States, in their work towards health for all, are continuing to formulate and implement national health strategies, of which plans for cancer control must form an increasingly important part. The WHO regional offices, and the WHO country representatives throughout the world, are providing valuable technical assistance for these initiatives.

In developing national cancer control programmes, it will be important for each country to create optimal conditions while undertaking a strategy development process for cancer control. These conditions include political will and commitment, collaboration among key national organizations, participatory processes in programme planning, critical assessment of the scientific evidence and costs of proposed programmes, and an approach based on maximizing the desired outcome, principally reduction in mortality from cancer. WHO can play a facilitating role with member countries that decide to develop or revise a national cancer control programme, by collaborating with them to advocate cancer control as a priority public health issue, by providing technical assistance during the development and implementation of cancer control guidelines, interventions and strategies, and by assisting with evaluation of programmes.

While this monograph provides guidance about what elements should be taken into account in establishing and maintaining national cancer control programmes, we are conscious that it does not provide comprehensive operational models for how to implement these recommendations. Although many countries will be able to successfully adapt the present guidelines to their particular situations, others, especially those with complex realities and constrained resources, will need further guidance in applying effective, operational methodologies for assuring adequate and sustainable performance of national cancer control programmes.

Considering this, and the suggestions from experts involved in revising this monograph, efforts will be made in the near future to develop a complementary volume that will focus on the "how", based on successful demonstration areas and specialized expertise. We are certain that such an initiative will be useful for those facing more challenging settings.

Cecilia Sepúlveda
Coordinator, Cancer Control Programme
World Health Organization
Geneva

EXECUTIVE SUMMARY

THIS MONOGRAPH outlines the scientific knowledge that is the basis for national cancer control programmes, and offers guidance on their establishment and organization. Much of its content derives from experience gained in the various countries that have already instituted or are planning their own national cancer control programmes.

Enough is now known about the causes of cancer and means of control for suitable interventions to have a significant impact. At least one-third of the 10 million new cases of cancer each year are preventable by such means as controlling tobacco and alcohol use, moderating diet, and immunizing against viral hepatitis B. Early detection, and therefore prompt treatment, of a further one-third of cases is possible where resources allow. Effective techniques are sufficiently well established to permit comprehensive palliative care for the remaining, more advanced, cases. The establishment of a national cancer control programme, tailored to the socioeconomic and cultural context, should allow countries to effectively and efficiently translate the present knowledge into action.

A national cancer control programme is a public health programme designed to reduce cancer incidence and mortality and improve quality of life of cancer patients, through the systematic and equitable implementation of evidence-based strategies for prevention, early detection, diagnosis, treatment, and palliation, making the best use of available resources.

The nature of cancer

The term cancer is used generically for more than 100 different diseases including malignant tumours of different sites (such as breast, cervix, prostate, stomach, colon/rectum, lung, mouth, leukaemia, sarcoma of bone, Hodgkin disease, and non-Hodgkin lymphoma). Common to all forms of the disease is the failure of the mechanisms that regulate normal cell growth, proliferation and cell death. Ultimately, there is progression of the resulting tumour from mild to severe abnormality, with invasion of neighbouring tissues and, eventually, spread to other areas of the body.

The disease arises principally as a consequence of exposure of individuals to carcinogenic (cancer-causing) agents in what they inhale, eat and drink, and are exposed to in their work or environment. Personal habits, such as tobacco use and dietary patterns, rather than inherited genetic factors, play the major roles in the etiology of cancer, as may occupational exposure to carcinogens and biological factors such as viral hepatitis B infection and human papillomavirus infection. Knowledge of many of these factors can serve as the basis of cancer control. Vaccination against hepatitis B, for instance, can protect against liver cancer.

Cancer is profoundly associated with social and economic status. Cancer risk factors are highest in groups with the least education. In addition, patients in the lower social classes have consistently poorer survival rates than those in the higher social classes.

The burden of cancer

Of the 10 million new cancer cases each year, 4.7 million are in the more developed countries and nearly 5.5 million are in the less developed countries. Although the disease has often been regarded principally as a problem of the developed world, in fact, more than half of all cancers occur in the developing countries. In developed countries, cancer is the second most common cause of death, and epidemiological evidence points to the emergence of a similar trend in developing countries.

Cancer is currently the cause of 12% of all deaths worldwide. In approximately 20 years time, the number of cancer deaths annually will increase from about 6 million to 10 million. The principal factors contributing to this projected increase are the increasing proportion of elderly people in the world (in whom cancer occurs more frequently than in the young), an overall decrease in deaths from communicable diseases, the decline in some countries in mortality from cardiovascular diseases, and the rising incidence of certain forms of cancer, notably lung cancer resulting from tobacco use. Approximately 20 million people are alive with cancer at present; by 2020 there will probably be more than 30 million.

The impact of cancer is far greater than the number of cases alone would suggest. Regardless of prognosis, the initial diagnosis of cancer is still perceived by many patients as a life-threatening event, with over one-third of patients experiencing clinical range anxiety and depression. Cancer can be equally if not more distressing for the family, profoundly affecting both the family's daily functioning and economic situation. The economic shock often includes both the loss of income and the expenses associated with health care costs.

Prevention of cancer

Prevention means eliminating or minimizing exposure to the causes of cancer, and includes reducing individual susceptibility to the effects of such causes. It is this approach that offers the greatest public health potential and the most cost-effective long-term cancer control.

The present and potential burden of tobacco-induced cancer is such that every country should give highest priority to tobacco control in its fight against cancer. Tobacco use in all forms is responsible for about 30% of all cancer deaths in developed countries, and this percentage is rising steadily in developing countries, particularly in women. The best approach to preventing tobacco-related cancer is preventing the uptake of tobacco. Tobacco dependence is listed in the WHO ICD-10 as a chronic condition. Tobacco is responsible for 80–90% of all lung cancer deaths, and probably some of the deaths from cancer of the oral cavity, larynx, oesophagus and stomach. In some Asian countries, oral cancer is a common tumour, and is associated with tobacco chewing habits. A comprehensive strategy involving legislative action to raise the tax on tobacco products and limit access and promotion, education of youth and adults to promote healthy life styles, and cessation programmes has a demonstrated ability to reduce tobacco consumption in many countries.

In recent years, substantial evidence has pointed to the link between overweight and obesity to many types of cancer such as oesophagus, colorectum, breast, endometrium and kidney. It is therefore strongly recommended to control weight and to avoid weight gain in adulthood by reducing caloric intake and by performing physical activity. The latter has also been seen to have a protective effect in reducing the risk of colorectal cancer. The composition of the diet is also important since fruit and vegetables might have a protective effect by decreasing the risk for some cancer types such as oral, oesophageal, gastric and colorectal cancer. High intake of preserved meat or red meat might be associated with increased risk of colorectal cancer. Another aspect of diet clearly related to cancer risk is the high consumption of alcoholic beverages, which convincingly increases the risk of cancer of the oral cavity, pharynx, larynx, oesophagus, liver and breast.

Thus, conducting a cancer prevention programme, within the context of an integrated noncommunicable disease prevention programme, is an effective national strategy. Tobacco use, alcohol, nutrition, physical inactivity, and obesity are risk factors common to other noncommunicable diseases, such as cardiovascular disease, diabetes, and respiratory diseases. Chronic disease prevention programmes can efficiently use the same surveillance and health promotion mechanisms.

Occupational and environmental exposure to a number of chemicals can cause cancer of a variety of sites; examples include lung cancer (asbestos), bladder cancer (aniline dyes), and leukaemia (benzene). A number of infections or infestations cause certain types of cancer: viral hepatitis B and C cause cancer of the liver, human papilloma virus infection causes cervical cancer, the bacterium *Helicobacter pylori* increases the risk of stomach cancer, while in some countries the parasitic infection schistosomiasis increases the risk of bladder cancer, and in other countries liver fluke infection increases the risk of cholangiocarcinoma of the bile ducts. Exposure to ionizing radiation is also known to give rise to certain cancers, and excessive solar ultraviolet radiation increases the risk of all types of cancer of the skin.

National policies and programmes can be enacted to reduce exposure to these risks and implement preventive interventions. Care needs to be taken to ensure that the public has a clear understanding of these major risks and is not overwhelmed by the minor risks that are described in their local media on a virtually daily basis.

Early detection of cancer

Early detection comprises early diagnosis in symptomatic populations and screening in asymptomatic, but at risk, populations. Increasing awareness of the signs and symptoms of cancer contributes to detection of the disease in less advanced stages. Where tests for cancer of specific sites are available, and facilities are appropriate, screening of apparently healthy individuals can disclose cancer in early or precursor stages, when treatment may be most effective. Early detection is only successful when linked to effective treatment.

With early detection, there is a greater chance that curative treatment will be successful, particularly for cancers of the breast, cervix, mouth, larynx, colon and rectum, and skin. It is therefore critical that people are taught to recognize early warning signs of the disease, such as lumps, sores that fail to heal, abnormal bleeding, persistent indigestion, and chronic hoarseness, and urged to seek prompt medical attention. This can be promoted in all countries by public health education campaigns and through training of primary health care workers.

Population screening (mass application of simple tests to identify individuals with asymptomatic disease) is another approach to early detection. However, screening programmes should be undertaken only when their effectiveness has been demonstrated, when resources (personnel, equipment and so on) are sufficient to cover nearly all of the target group, when facilities exist for confirming diagnoses and for treatment and follow-up of those with abnormal results, and when prevalence of the disease is high enough to justify the effort and costs of screening. At present, in countries with high levels of resources, screening can be advocated only for cancer of the breast and cervix. Efforts should concentrate on women at greatest risk of developing invasive cancer: those aged 35 years and over for cervical cancer and those aged over 50 years for breast cancer. In developing countries, organized screening should only be considered for cervical cancer and should focus primarily on providing a limited number of screenings with maximum population coverage, because the women at greatest risk for cervical cancer are in general the last to approach the health care services.

Diagnosis and treatment of cancer

Cancer diagnosis is the first step to cancer management. This calls for a combination of careful clinical assessment and diagnostic investigations including endoscopy, imaging, hystopathology, cytology and laboratory studies. Once a diagnosis is confirmed, it is necessary to ascertain cancer staging, where the main goals are to aid in the choice of therapy, prognostication, and to standardize the design of research treatment protocols.

The primary objectives of cancer treatment are cure, prolongation of life, and improvement of the quality of life. A national cancer control programme should therefore establish guidelines for integrating treatment resources with programmes for early detection, and provide therapeutic standards for the most important cancers in the country.

Care of cancer patients typically starts with recognition of an abnormality, followed by consultation at a health care facility with appropriate services for diagnosis and treatment. Treatment may involve surgery, radiation therapy, chemotherapy, hormonal therapy, or some combination of these. An initial priority, especially in developing countries, should be the development of national diagnostic and treatment guidelines to establish a minimum standard of care, and promote the rational use of existing resources and greater equity in access to treatment services.

Optimal treatment of people diagnosed with certain types of cancer detected early, for example, cancers of the uterine cervix and corpus, breast, testis, and melanoma, will result in 5-year survival rates of 75% or more. By contrast, survival rates in patients with cancer of the pancreas, liver, stomach, and lung are generally less than 15%. Some treatments require sophisticated technology that is available only in locations with substantial resources. Since the cost of establishing and maintaining such facilities is high, it is desirable that they should initially be concentrated in relatively few places in a country to avoid draining resources that could be devoted to other aspects of the national cancer control programme. Facilities can be expanded when additional resources are available.

Palliative care

Palliative care is an approach that improves the quality of life of patients and their families facing the problems associated with life-threatening illness, through the prevention and relief of suffering by means of early identification and impeccable assessment and treatment of pain and other problems, physical, psychosocial and spiritual.

Improved quality of life is of paramount importance to patients with cancer. Pain relief and palliative care must therefore be regarded as integral and essential elements of a national cancer control programme, whatever the possibilities of cure. Since these services can be provided relatively simply and inexpensively, they should be available in every country and should be given high priority, especially in developing countries where cure of the majority of cancer patients is likely to remain beyond reach for years to come.

Health workers and family care givers can be trained to deliver palliative care effectively. Primary health care settings can respond to the majority of patients' needs and, in many developing countries with poor infrastructure, home-based care will make an essential contribution to achieving the necessary coverage.

Effective guidelines for the relief of cancer pain and other symptoms have been developed by WHO. The WHO ladder for cancer pain relief is a key strategy for pain management that can relieve cancer pain for about 90% of patients. Analgesics are administered by mouth, using a three-step strategy of strengthening the analgesic when a lower level is insufficient to relieve pain, and medication is provided by the clock, rather than waiting for the effect of the previous dose to have fully worn off. The widespread availability of morphine for oral administration is critical to pain relief, and should be ensured by appropriate legislation and policy.

Managing national cancer control programmes

With careful planning and appropriate priorities, within the scope of prevention, early detection, treatment and palliation, the establishment of national cancer control programmes offers the most rational means of achieving a substantial degree of cancer control, even where resources are severely limited. It is for this reason that the establishment of a national cancer control programme is recommended wherever the burden of the disease is significant, there is a rising trend of cancer risk factors and there is a need to make the most efficient use of limited resources.

Effective and efficient cancer control programmes need competent management to identify priorities and resources (planning), and to organize and coordinate those resources to guarantee sustained progress to meet the planned objectives (implementation, monitoring and evaluation). Good management is essential to maintain momentum and introduce any necessary modifications. A quality management approach is essential to improving the performance of the programme. Such an approach has the following principles:

- *goal orientation* that continuously guides the processes towards improving the health and quality of life of the people covered by the programme.
- *focused on the needs of the people*, which implies focusing on the target population (customers) while addressing the needs of all stakeholders and ensuring their active involvement.
- *systematic decision making process*, based on evidence, social values, and efficient use of resources that benefits the majority of the target population.
- *systemic and comprehensive approach*, meaning that the programme is a comprehensive system with interrelated key components in the different levels of care sharing the same goal, integrated with other programmes and the health system and tailored to the social context, rather than a vertical programme operating in isolation.
- *leadership* that creates a clarity and unity of purpose, encourages team building, ample participation, ownership of the process, continuous learning, and mutual recognition of efforts made.
- *partnership*, enhancing effectiveness through mutually beneficial relationships, built on trust and complementary capacities, with partners from different disciplines and sectors.
- *continual improvement, innovation and creativity*, to maximize performance, and to address social and cultural diversity, and the new needs and challenges in a changing environment.

The motivation to initiate a national cancer control programme or improve the performance of an existing programme can come from different sectors within the country or can be a combined effort with international organizations. Governmental and nongovernmental leaders in the cancer field need to work closely together to develop a successful programme. With appropriate mobilization of all the stakeholders, it is possible to develop cancer control policies that are acceptable to the people for whom they are intended, affordable, integrated with other national health programmes, and linked effectively with sectors other than health that are relevant to cancer control.

Although it is clear that objectives and priorities need to be tailored to the specific country context, the planning processes to be undertaken in all countries should follow four basic steps: assessing the magnitude of the cancer problem, setting measurable control objectives, evaluating possible strategies for cancer prevention and control, and choosing priorities for initial cancer control activities. Assessing the magnitude of the cancer problem requires analysis of the cancer burden and risk factors, as well as capacity assessment (analysis of facilities, personnel, programmes and services). Once evidence-based strategies are identified there is the need to choose those that are feasible to implement and that are acceptable and relevant to the society. It is useful to classify priority areas in two groups: activities that can be introduced or improved without the need for additional resources, and activities that will require extra resources.

The national cancer control programme policy should be formulated once the planning process has been completed. This will provide a solid platform for implementing and maintaining a national cancer control programme. A policy is the explicit commitment by government and its partners that provides objectives for a balanced cancer control programme, specifies the relative priority of each objective and indicates the resources and measures required to attain the objectives.

Good leadership of the programme is key to its competent management. The national programme coordinator should be able to work in a team and facilitate or reinforce the building of a network of local coordinators, backed by their own teams, who will take a leadership role in their areas or regions. It is essential to build effective teams, that are results oriented and committed to the project objectives, goals and strategies, as most of the managerial, clinical or community activities in a cancer control programme require teamwork

Processes should be managed to meet the requirements and needs of customers, providers and other stakeholders. Clear roles and responsibilities must be established for managing the process and the interrelations with other programmes must be identified. The processes must align with the national cancer control programme objectives and should include continual improvement of performance. Decisions and actions should be based on the analysis of data and information to improve results and not rely merely on opinions.

Some key processes to be considered in implementing a national cancer control programme are:

Demonstration area

It is often advisable to start small and consider that success breeds success. Efforts can concentrate in a demonstration area, which has a good likelihood of successfully implementing the priority areas.

Step by step implementation

Implementation of a national cancer control programme may proceed in a series of stages, each stage having clear measurable objectives and representing the basis for the development of the next stage, permitting visible and controlled progress. Every stage should involve decision-makers and operational staff from the different levels of care that need to actively participate.

Optimizing existing resources

It is essential that at a first stage the programme considers re-allocation of existing resources according to the new strategies, and foresees the development and incorporation of new technologies that are cost-effective, sustainable and of benefit to the majority of the targeted population.

Organizing activities with a systemic approach

Activities carried out according to the selected priorities should be tailored to the population at risk and adequately organized so as to make the best use of the available resources. Furthermore, it is important to take a systemic approach to ensure that the various interrelated components of the intervention strategy are coordinated, directed to achieving the objectives and integrated with other related programmes or initiatives.

Education and training

Programmes to educate and train health care professionals, customers, and other stakeholders should be tailored to the type of audience, to the local situation and the momentum in the programme development so as to ensure that they can contribute to improving the programme.

Monitoring and evaluation

Evaluation activities can be seen as part of a continuum that supports the decision-making process in all stages of programming: planning, implementation and outcome evaluation. Continuous evaluation of national cancer control programme processes (monitoring) and outcomes should be considered an essential tool for assessing its organizational progress and enhancing its effectiveness.

Programme monitoring is intended to assess whether a national cancer control programme is performing as intended, and whether or not the programme is reaching the target population and meeting the needs of customers. Programme performance can be assessed by different methods, depending on how comprehensive an evaluation is required and which quality dimensions are of interest (effectiveness, efficiency, competence, appropriateness, accessibility, and so on). *Outcome indicators* for a national cancer control programme are concerned with the quality of life of cancer patients, disease recurrence rates, disease-free survival rates, overall survival rates among treated patients, incidence, and mortality rates. Reliable baseline data on the common types of cancer, their stage at diagnosis, and the outcome of disease are essential if valid programme outcome measures are to be set. Evaluation is completely dependent on adequate information systems that should be developed as early in the programme as possible in order to monitor processes and indicate changes to improve them. They should be linked to population-based cancer registries in the areas where they exist so that outcome measures can be provided by the surveillance system.

National cancer control activities
based on resource realities

Some of the previously described cancer control strategies may be far beyond the resources of many countries. Nevertheless, there is a clear benefit in implementing a national cancer control programme, regardless of the fiscal situation in a country. The programme process will ensure the most efficient use of existing resources in the control of cancer.

In general, the majority of cancer patients in developing countries are diagnosed at advanced stages of the disease, because of the lack of awareness of the need for rapid action if a cancer symptom or sign is detected, the lack of early detection programmes, and the limited resources for diagnosis and treatment. However, developing countries do not constitute a homogeneous group. Important differences can be encountered with regard to the epidemiological situation, and to economic, social and health system development. The various settings need to be taken into account when addressing the cancer problem and organizing a programme at the national or state level. Further, there are often large social inequalities within a specific country. While a considerable proportion of the population of a developing country will be poor and face major barriers to social development, in contrast a small percentage is likely to be wealthy and in many cases to enjoy a standard of living and health level comparable to those in developed countries.

A flexible approach is needed, as political, socioeconomic and epidemiological situations vary and evolve. With this in mind, three separate scenarios are provided to help guide countries toward what is possible with their limited level of resources (low, medium or high). As well as being relevant to individual countries, the scenarios can be used to identify specific actions relevant to regions or different population groups within a country.

Low level of resources (Scenario A)

This scenario refers to low income countries where resources for chronic disease are completely absent or very limited. Many such countries may have great political and social instability. A considerable proportion of the population is rural. Infant and adult mortality rates are high. Communicable diseases and malnutrition are a major cause of morbidity and mortality, especially for children. Life expectancy is relatively low. Cancer is not one of the main problems in general, but over 15 years of age it can be one of the leading causes of death. The majority of cancer patients are diagnosed in advanced stages. Exposure to cancer risk factors such as tobacco or environmental carcinogens other than aflatoxin may be low but almost invariably rising. Exposure to infectious causes of cancer will usually be high (human papillomaviruses and hepatitis B virus, and sometimes schistosomiasis). Health care services are often delivered by informal means, and alternative medicine is a major component. Infrastructure and human resources for cancer prevention or control are non-existent or very limited in quantity, quality and accessibility.

What can be done in such circumstances? The first immediate action is to establish a basis for prevention of cancer and other chronic diseases by limiting the extent to which the health scourges of the industrialized world – tobacco use and the "western diet" – can enter the country. There are already enough health problems within the country without importing those from outside. The general public and health care workers can be made aware of the early warning signs of cancer and other diseases. This will ensure that cases are identified, referred and treated early in the course of disease, before they become advanced and incurable. The process of establishing national diagnosis and treatment guidelines has the dual purpose of determining effective patient management standards as well as promoting equitable access to the limited treatment resources. Perhaps the most significant contribution of a national cancer control programme in this scenario is establishing a basis for pain relief and palliative care of individuals with advanced disease to ensure that they maintain a high as possible quality of life. Allocation of available resources in a cost-effective manner is of greatest concern in areas with a low level of resources, and is assured by the quantitative-based strategy evaluation process of establishing a national cancer control programme.

Medium level of resources (Scenario B)

Countries in this scenario are often considered "middle-income" countries. The majority of the population is urban and life expectancy is over 60 years. The country has been through the epidemiological transition, and cancer is usually one of the leading causes of disease and mortality. There is a high exposure to risk factors, especially tobacco, diet, infectious agents, and carcinogens in the workplace. Infrastructure and human resources for developing cancer prevention, early detection, diagnosis, treatment, and palliative care are available but with limitations in quantity, quality, and accessibility. Weaknesses can be identified in organization, priority setting, resource allocation, and information systems for adequate monitoring and evaluation. Primary prevention and early detection are usually neglected in favour of treatment-oriented approaches, without much concern regarding their cost-effectiveness.

In general, the primary prevention activities needed in this type of setting are tobacco control, reduction of alcohol use, and promotion of healthy diet and physical exercise. Special attention should be paid to carcinogens in the workplace, and to infectious agents such as human papilloma virus. Promotion of the warning signs for the common cancers should be encouraged. If, as is common in this scenario, rates of cervical cancer are high, the highest priority for a screening programme is cervical cytology screening, focusing mainly on covering a high proportion of the women at risk. Screening for other types of cancers should be discouraged. Cancer treatment should focus on cancers that are curable, and clinical trials should be encouraged to evaluate relatively low-cost approaches that eventually can be provided to all patients irrespective of their socioeconomic condition. More sophisticated approaches, such as radiotherapy and chemotherapy, should be introduced in specialized centres. Major efforts should be made to achieve the highest coverage for pain relief and palliative care, using low cost drugs (oral morphine) and other interventions.

High level of resources (Scenario C)

This scenario is appropriate for industrialized countries with a relatively high level of resources for health care. In these countries life expectancy is over 70 years, and cancer is a major cause of death for both men and women. Many elements of a cancer control programme are in place, but they may not be well integrated into a comprehensive national system. Further, coverage of the population may be uneven, with particular groups such as those in rural areas, indigenous people and recent immigrants having difficulty accessing services. Reorganization of the system could bring benefits in terms of greater cost effectiveness and improved reach and acceptability of services.

Comprehensive health promotion programmes, including in schools and workplaces, should be implemented in collaboration with other sectors. While there should be a concerted effort to promote awareness of the early warning signs for cancer, national screening programmes should, in general, only be implemented for cervical and breast cancer, as screening for other cancers has not yet been proven to be cost-effective. In spite of a high level of resources, industrialized countries often have serious deficiencies with respect to providing easy access to pain relief and palliative care services. Implementation of a comprehensive surveillance system ensures rapid response to changes in disease patterns and weaknesses in service provision.

Knowledge gained over the past decades provides enormous scope for controlling cancer throughout the world, and the most appropriate mechanism for exploiting that knowledge is through the establishment of national cancer control programmes.

The recommendations for minimum essential actions by national cancer control programmes, in countries with different levels of resources, are summarized in Table 13.1. A more detailed coverage of these recommendations is provided in Chapter 13.

Challenges Facing Cancer Control Programmes

THE AIM OF CANCER CONTROL is a reduction in incidence and mortality of cancer as well as an improvement in the quality of life of cancer patients and their families. This requires sound knowledge of the carcinogenesis process and the factors that influence the course of the disease, and an understanding of the social, economic and organizational factors that govern how that knowledge can be put to effective use. The word "control" does not imply that cancer can be eradicated in the way that an infectious disease can be eradicated by immunization, but rather that control can be exercised over its causes and consequences. The concept of cancer control empowers society to achieve mastery over the disease.

The magnitude of the cancer problem, and its growing importance in almost all countries, coupled with the knowledge now available, are compelling reasons for the development of national strategies for cancer control.

Chapter 1 deals with the biological and social aspects of the group of diseases known as cancer. Chapter 2 considers the causes of cancer and their relative importance in terms of public health. Chapter 3 reviews cancer patterns and trends, and their socioeconomic impact.

BIOLOGICAL AND SOCIAL ASPECTS OF CANCER

1

BIOLOGICAL ASPECTS
OF CANCER

Cancer is the generic term for a group of diseases that can affect any part of the body. Malignant tumours of the brain, lung, breast, prostate, skin, and colon are among the diseases known as cancer. Other examples of cancers include leukaemia, sarcomas, Hodgkin disease and non-Hodgkin lymphoma. Certain common morphological features differentiate all forms of cancer from other types of disease, including other noncommunicable diseases and diseases caused by toxic agents. Yet there are links between cancer and these other diseases. In particular many noncommunicable diseases share causal factors, such as tobacco use, unhealthy diet, obesity, and lack of physical exercise. Approaches to prevention are therefore often identical.

Cancers share several biological characteristics. One defining feature is the proliferation of abnormal cells. The process of cell turnover is normally well controlled throughout life by basic biological mechanisms. In cancer, however, the control mechanisms go awry. Cells in the affected part of the body grow beyond their usual boundaries, invade adjoining tissues, and may spread to secondary organs or tissues as metastases.

Advances in molecular biology have improved researchers' understanding of the mechanisms of normal cell growth, making it possible to investigate the aberrant cell proliferation and failure of programmed cell death (apoptosis) that constitute cancer. Cell growth is under the control of a class of genes known as the proto-oncogenes or suppressor genes. If gene mutation or translocation occurs within a chromosome, a proto-oncogene may lose its capacity to regulate cell replication and become an oncogene. Such genetic changes, triggered by a variety of factors, may constitute the final common pathway in the biological mechanism of cancer.

A malignant tumour originates from one altered cell and initially proliferates at the primary site. Subsequently, it usually spreads through various pathways, such as by local infiltration in the neighbourhood of the organ of origin, lymphatic system (lymph nodes) or the vascular channels, leading to metastasis. Metastases are the major cause of death from malignant diseases.

Phases in the development of cancer

Cancer develops in several phases, depending on the type of tissue affected. Typically, these phases are: dysplasia, cancer *in situ*, localized invasive cancer, regional lymph node involvement, and distant metastases (see Figure 1.1).

The first indication of abnormality is a change in the character of cells, known as dysplasia. The lesion may regress spontaneously at this stage, and sometimes even at the next, carcinoma *in situ* (as indicated by the arrows in both directions). The term "carcinoma *in situ*" is used when microscopic examination discloses cells with certain characteristics of cancer, that is, changes in the cell nuclei, but with no penetration of the underlying (or basement) membrane that holds them in the tissue of origin. The term carcinoma *in situ* is usually reserved for changes that affect the full thickness of the epithelium.

When the abnormal cell growth reaches areas underlying the tissue of origin, the cancer is regarded as invasive. With further growth, there is increasing invasion and destruction of adjacent tissues. Often, the cancer extends to the regional lymph nodes that drain the area. Cancer cells may also spread through the blood or lymphatic system to affect other organs (distant metastases). For example, cancer in the colon may spread to the liver or lungs.

With sufficient multiplication of abnormal cells, the cancer becomes apparent to the individual or to the physician. It commonly takes the form of a lump that may be seen or felt in the organ involved, for example skin, breast, or prostate. Sometimes, even before detection, the cancer will have spread to lymph nodes or, if rapidly progressive, will have already caused detectable distant metastases. The growth of the cancer can involve blood vessels and cause bleeding, which will be apparent if the cancer reaches part of an organ

Fig. 1.1 Typical phases of cancer development

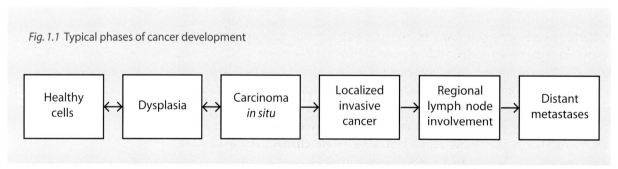

that is in direct or indirect contact with the exterior. For example, there may be blood in the sputum from lung cancer, blood in the stools from bowel cancer, or blood in the urine from bladder cancer. The growth of a cancer may also cause functional disturbances: for example, cancer of the brain may give rise to neurological symptoms and signs. In advanced cancer, one of the most severe symptoms is the pain induced by pressure on nerves.

Implications of biology for cancer control

The genetic changes that characterize cancer sometimes occur as a consequence of defective hereditary material. However, hereditary forms of cancer are relatively rare, and more commonly the relevant genetic changes take place as a result of an external influence.

One approach to preventing cancers is to identify the external agents and factors responsible for the cell changes that lead to cancer. Certain chemicals, for example, are known to be carcinogenic; that is, they induce the cellular changes characteristic of cancer. Controlling exposure to such chemicals, or to complex mixtures (such as tobacco smoke) that contain many carcinogens, may, therefore, prevent some cancers. Interfering with the transmission of an infectious agent such as a virus may prevent other cancers. Still other cancers may be prevented by using an agent that directly interferes with the carcinogenic process – an approach termed chemoprevention.

Even after the malignancy has started, it may still be possible to prevent progression to the invasive form of the disease. Techniques have been developed to detect the early phases of certain cancers, notably those of the uterine cervix, before symptoms are manifest. Timely recognition and excision of dysplasia or *in situ* cancer can prevent the progression to invasive cancer. Even when cancer has become invasive, arrest or cure can be effected in some cases by removing cancer surgically or destroying the cancer cells by radiation or chemotherapy.

SOCIAL ASPECTS OF CANCER

Cancer arises largely as a result of lifestyle, and is thus a consequence of the conditions in which individuals live and work. For some cancers, specific causal relationships to chemicals are well established; leukaemia as a result of exposure to benzene used in tyre manufacture is one example. Lifestyle influences are relevant for most cancers. The changes in incidence of different forms of cancer among migrants who have moved from one part of the world to another probably reflects major lifestyle changes resulting from acculturation to the way of life in the host country.

Where people live

A striking feature of cancer is its geographical and temporal variability. The population of a particular place at a specific time exhibits a certain pattern of cancer, with more cases of one type and fewer of another. In another place, or at another time, the pattern of cancer in the population will be different. This is illustrated by the following examples.

The incidence of liver cancer in sub-Saharan Africa and south-east Asia is high compared with that in western Europe. During the early part of the twentieth century, residents of North America and Europe suffered only rarely from lung cancer, but succeeding generations living in the same areas have experienced a lung cancer epidemic because of the widespread adoption of cigarette smoking. This epidemic is now expanding rapidly to Asia as a consequence of Asians increasingly taking up the smoking habits of the West.

Stomach cancer is significantly more common among the people of Chile, northern China, Japan, and the countries of eastern Europe than among those living in other parts of the world. These differences are probably largely attributable to changes in dietary patterns and means of food preservation, although differences in the prevalence of infection with the bacterium *Helicobacter pylori* may also be a contributory factor. Social aspects are, however, also evident: the incidence of stomach cancer among people of low socioeconomic status is greater than among those who are more socially advantaged.

In a few rare cases, the location in which people live may give rise to cancer. This is true of certain parts of Turkey, where the incidence of mesothelioma is extremely high because people live where the earth's crust is composed of erionite, an asbestiform material (Artvinli and Baris, 1979). Exposure during early life appears to lead to the disease decades later.

Changes people make in the world

Wherever people settle, part of the way they adapt to prevailing conditions is to exploit the earth for its resources. This may expose them to cancer-causing agents or influences not previously encountered. Industrial workers have suffered most severely. For example, more than half of certain groups of miners who worked in the Joachimsthal and Schneeburg mines of central Europe during the latter part of the nineteenth century died of lung cancer, a rare disease at that time, as a result of exposure to radioactivity in the mines.

The manufacture of dyestuffs can also lead to cancer. The manufacture and use of 2-naphthylamine, for example, causes bladder cancer. Exposure to 2-naphthylamine was at first concentrated in North America and Europe. It has now largely ceased there, only to reappear in southern Asia. Industrial development has often exported risks to areas where local people do not recognize those risks.

Implications of lifestyle for cancer control

Human existence is characterized by behaviour patterns—what people do to meet their biological, psychological, and social needs. These patterns may include certain ways of preparing and consuming food, physical inactivity, and the development of dependence on tobacco products, alcohol, and drugs. Many of these patterns have an impact on cancer, as well as on other diseases. Adopting a healthy lifestyle that includes a healthy diet, physical exercise, appropriate body weight, and avoidance of risk-associated behaviours can lead to a long active life.

Social and economic inequities

Cancer and other chronic diseases are profoundly associated with social and economic status. Tobacco use, displacement of vegetables and fruit by high-fat/low-fibre foods, reduced physical activity, and alcohol abuse are highest in groups with the least education (Yach, 2001). For example, as shown in Figure 1.2, for females in Bombay, India, the lower the educational level, the higher the proportion of tobacco use (Gupta, 1996). Poorer groups are often explicitly targeted in the marketing of unhealthy products, and are also the least likely to be reached by preventive and promotion measures.

Primary health care services have always focused on acute care for infants and mothers, rather than evolving to deal with the rising rates of cancer and other noncommunicable diseases. The consequences of limited access to health services are evident in reduced survival rates and more pain for cancer patients. Patients in the lower social classes have consistently poorer survival rates than those in the higher social classes. Social class is associated with access to care. For cancer patients, access to care is in turn associated with survival and quality of life.

Strategies for cancer control must take into account the limitations imposed, as well as the opportunities created, by the social aspects of the problem. Understanding how particular features of people's social circumstances and development contribute to cancer can point the way to avoiding or correcting the socioeconomic factors that are mainly responsible for the disease.

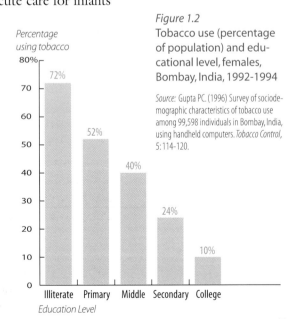

Figure 1.2
Tobacco use (percentage of population) and educational level, females, Bombay, India, 1992-1994

Source: Gupta PC. (1996) Survey of sociodemographic characteristics of tobacco use among 99,598 individuals in Bombay, India, using handheld computers. *Tobacco Control,* 5: 114-120.

CAUSES OF CANCER

2

BIOLOGICAL AND GENETIC FACTORS

The cellular changes that characterize cancer are initiated by various degrees of interaction between host factors and exogenous agents.

Although host factors other than genes play a role in the development of the disease, some of these are increasingly being recognized as also being under genetic influence. These include hormonal patterns and immunological capacities. The common cancers of sex-specific organs – especially the uterus, breast, ovary and prostate – are influenced by levels of sex hormones. There is a positive link, for example, between breast cancer and elevated levels of the hormone estradiol. Suppression of immunological function, such as that required following organ transplantation or occurring in acquired immunodeficiency syndrome (AIDS), enhances the incidence of certain lymphomas and perhaps other cancers.

Genetics and cancer

Cancer occurs because of mutations in the genes responsible for cell multiplication and repair. This does not mean that the disease is heritable. Indeed, it now seems clear that even the rare so-called heritable cancers caused by genes of high penetrance, and transmitted through Mendelian laws, mostly require a particular interaction with environmental factors for induction. Although the distinction between high and low penetrance genes obscures a continuum of susceptibility at the biological level, it is possible at the operational level to identify a small number of genes (high penetrance genes) in which pathological mutations are sufficiently predictive of cancer risk to influence clinical management. In contrast, any allelic variant of the "major" genes, or alteration in other interactive genes or in environmentally sensitive polymorphisms that would not be sufficiently penetrant to affect clinical practice, is categorized as low penetrance. Nevertheless, as knowledge expands and the capacity to test multiple genes simultaneously becomes commonplace, high penetrance "genotypes" comprising several low penetrance genetic variations may be recognized.

Genetics may therefore eventually play an important role in the control of cancer, including:

- identification of individuals at risk for a specific cancer, leading to preventive or screening strategies for an individual or family members;
- identification of cancer subtype so that treatment can be tailored to target that specific disease.

The potential role of genetics should not, however, be overstated. Studies have shown that the primary determinants of most cancers are lifestyle factors, such as tobacco, dietary and exercise habits, and infectious agents, rather than inherited genetic factors. For example, probably only 5% of all breast cancers occur in women with a genetic predisposition to the disease.

At present, the major practical role for cancer genetics is the identification of individuals at high risk for cancer. Information on the history of cancer in a family should be routinely collected in all countries. Routine DNA-based genetic testing for high penetrance genes (such as BRCA 1 or 2 for breast cancer) is currently only feasible in some of the most affluent countries.

Family history and DNA screening can identify individuals at moderately increased risk of cancer and individuals from cancer-prone families. Identification of such people allows them to make informed decisions regarding reproduction, lifestyle and clinical risk-reduction strategies. When genetic information indicates an increased risk of a cancer, those at risk may undergo more intensive or more frequent early detection interventions than are routine, in an attempt to detect a cancer at a more treatable stage.

While cancer-prone families are quite rare, the risk of a specific cancer within such a family can be very high. Genetic testing of a person with cancer can help clarify the risk to offspring. It can also serve as the basis for subsequent genetic counselling of the offspring or family, with a view to increasing their understanding of the medical situation and encouraging them to adopt strategies to minimize subsequent cancer risk.

In practice, the type of high risk genetic susceptibility caused by high penetrance genes transmitted in a Mendelian fashion is uncommon, and the proportion of cancers caused by such predisposition is low (about 5% for breast or colon cancer and less for most other cancers, except for retinoblastoma in children). In contrast, it is now appreciated that so-called metabolic polymorphisms, that is differences in the way people metabolize chemical carcinogens, can explain differences in the susceptibility of individuals to cancer, and that these polymorphisms are controlled at a cellular level by mutations in specific genes. A major research endeavour is now under way to characterize these genetic polymorphisms. It is already clear that there are multiplicities of such genetic changes, that they are caused by genes of low penetrance, and that the classic Mendelian laws of inheritance do not apply. However, it seems likely that collectively these polymorphisms explain much of the innate susceptibility to cancer, and that consequently their potential contribution to the occurrence of cancer is large. Furthermore, interactions with environmental factors seem to be frequently associated with genetic changes. Thus it may be eventually possible to identify those individuals at special risk of tobacco or diet-associated cancers, and also those susceptible to the effects of environmental contaminants.

It is also anticipated, but not yet proven, that genetic testing may eventually provide information that will be used to determine the best course of treatment for some cancers. Certain cancers currently classified as a single disease may ultimately be classified into different types, each best managed by a different therapeutic strategy. Beyond the drawback of the high costs of genetic testing, there are also potential problems associated with patient privacy and discrimination. Who should have access to genetic information and for what purposes should such information be used? The potential for discrimination regarding employment and access to health insurance is considerable. Safeguards against inappropriate use are, however, being developed. If the full potential of the human genome project is to be realized, it is important to avoid erecting barriers that will block the potential advances in cancer prevention, diagnosis and therapy that might be achieved through such testing.

EXTERNAL AGENTS

The wealth of current knowledge about the influence of external environmental determinants of cancer provides significant potential for cancer control. These external factors can be categorized as follows:

- *physical*, for example, solar radiation (which can give rise to skin cancer), and ionizing radiation (which induces cancer of the lung and certain other organs);
- *chemical*, for example, vinyl chloride (which can cause liver cancer), 2-naphthylamine, (which can cause cancer of the bladder), and benzopyrene (which can cause tobacco-related cancers);
- *biological*, for example, hepatitis B virus (which is a cause of liver cancer), and human papilloma virus (which is a cause of cancer of the cervix).

Cancer typically arises many years after initial contact with the etiological agent. For example, exposure to asbestos can result in the development of mesothelioma several decades later.

A dose-response gradient generally governs the development of cancer following exposure to a carcinogen. The greater the extent of exposure, the more likely it is that the disease will occur. Thus, people who lived close to the centre of the atomic blast in Hiroshima were exposed to higher radiation levels and suffered greater incidence of various forms of cancer than people who lived towards the periphery of the affected area (Kato and Schull, 1982).

Carcinogenic risks, though encountered almost universally, are not the same in all parts of the world. In developed countries, for example, the extensive use of X-rays for diagnostic and therapeutic purposes is generally well accepted, even though the radiation may contribute to the development of certain types of cancer, especially leukaemia. In the same countries, food-handling methods—another lifestyle factor—minimize accumulation of the mould that produces aflatoxin, which is a liver carcinogen (IARC, 1993). In many African countries, by contrast, there is little or no danger from medical X-radiation, but people continue to store food under conditions that favour the production of aflatoxin.

Physical carcinogens

Both ionizing and non-ionizing radiation can cause cancer. Small amounts of ionizing radiation occur naturally, specifically in cosmic rays and in radioactive materials in the earth. Exposure may thus result from this "background" radiation, from medical and occupational contact with radiation, from accidents at nuclear power stations, or from the use of nuclear weapons in war. Some types of leukaemia and cancers of the breast, lung, and thyroid are specifically associated with exposure to ionizing radiation. However, ionizing radiation may also increase the likelihood of cancer of most other sites, including the stomach, large intestine, and bladder. Ionizing radiation does not, however, increase the likelihood of chronic lymphatic leukaemia.

Exposure to non-ionizing ultraviolet radiation in sunlight gives rise to the common forms of skin cancer in Caucasian populations (IARC, 1992). Burning from solar radiation is associated with the rarer, but more fatal, melanoma. Individuals with light complexions are especially at risk.

Certain materials have physical properties that are the cause of a number of forms of cancer. In the case of asbestos, for example, the length and toughness of the constituent fibres seems to be important in causing lung cancer, mesothelioma and probably cancer of the larynx, as well as many forms of gastrointestinal cancer.

Chemical carcinogens

Extensive evidence of chemical carcinogenesis has come from studies of people whose occupations bring them into contact with various substances (Table 4.2). Excessive alcohol use (IARC, 1988), and certain drugs (IARC, 1996) also increase the risk of some cancers. Vaginal cancer among young women was found to be due to diethylstilbestrol, a synthetic hormone that had been given to their mothers to prevent miscarriage during pregnancy (Lanier et al., 1973). Overshadowing all these, however, is the critical role of tobacco smoking as a leading cause of cancer in many countries (IARC, 1986).

Biological carcinogens

Examples of cancer caused by living organisms include bladder cancer resulting from infection with the parasite *Schistosoma haematobium* (IARC, 1994a), liver cancer following viral hepatitis B and C infection (IARC, 1994b), gastric cancer following infection with *Helicobacter pylori* (IARC,1994a) and cancer of the uterine cervix following human papillomavirus infection (IARC, 1995).

Dietary factors

Several studies indicate that vegetables and fruits contain substances that provide protection against some cancers. Similarly, studies indicate that excessive amounts of animal products in the diet, such as red meat, increase the risk of colorectal and perhaps breast cancer and other forms of the disease (World Cancer Research Fund, American Institute for Cancer Research, 1997). Among the diet related factors overweight/obesity convincingly increases the risk of several common cancers such as colorectal and breast cancer (Joint WHO/FAO expert consultation on diet, nutrition and the prevention of chronic diseases, in preparation).

Occupation

The impetus for identifying occupationally-induced cancers has come from three principal factors:
- increased competence in recognizing and demonstrating occupational hazards;
- social pressures;
- the growing diversity of industrial processes and the concomitant exposure of workers to physical and chemical carcinogens.

Among the industries in which there is evidence of carcinogenic risk are the following: agriculture, construction, demolition, shipbuilding, shipbreaking, petroleum, metal and rubber (Tomatis et al., 1990; IARC, 1990).

Development of an effective strategy for the prevention of occupationally-induced cancers requires detailed knowledge of which exposures carry significant risk. The aim of the strategy will then be to modify or, if necessary, abandon certain operations so as to reduce or eliminate those risks.

Air and water pollution

Throughout the world, carcinogenic agents are released into the air and into surface and ground waters as a result of industrial processes and the accidental or deliberate dumping of toxic wastes. According to current evidence, however, these relatively common forms of pollution seem to be less significant than lifestyle factors in causing cancer. A small number of people are at high risk of exposure to carcinogenic pollutants, but for most the risk is minor and difficult to quantify. Verification of a cause/effect relationship in the latter case would involve measuring the exposure of very large numbers of people and then observing them to determine the consequences of exposure (Committee on Environmental Epidemiology, 1991).

The role of medical services and care

Although rare, some incidences of cancer have been iatrogenically induced. For example, routine use of X-ray fluoroscopy to follow the course of tuberculosis induced breast cancer in some patients (Miller et al., 1989). Further, some drugs used to treat cancer are carcinogenic, while estrogens – used to counteract menopausal symptoms – increase the risk of endometrial and breast cancer (IARC, 1999). It is essential, therefore, to carefully weigh up the benefits of these methods against the risks inherent in their use.

RELATIVE IMPORTANCE OF VARIOUS CAUSES OF CANCER

Cancer of the oral cavity, which is the commonest form of the disease in much of south-east Asia, accounts for half the total incidence of cancer in some parts of India, with 90% of cases attributable to smoking or chewing tobacco (Tomatis et al., 1990). A quarter of all cancer deaths in North America are from lung cancer, and 80-90% of these are the result of cigarette smoking. Table 2.1 shows the estimated percentages of cancer deaths attributable to various causes in people under the age of 65 years in the United States of America. These estimates probably apply to most industrialized countries, although the figures may well underestimate the proportion of cancers caused by occupational factors, many of which become apparent only after workers have retired. Recent evidence suggests that the proportion of cancers related to diet is less than 35%, although a definitive value is not yet available. Diet-related factors are now thought to account for about

30% of cancers in developed countries and perhaps 20% of cancers in developing countries. Infectious agents may account for about 15% of cancers in the world. The vast majority of these cases occur in developing countries where communicable diseases are much more prevalent. There would be 21% fewer cases of cancer in developing countries and 9% fewer cases in developed countries if these cancer related infectious diseases were prevented (Pisani et al., 1997).

With regard to occupational risks, one estimate for Canada was that 9% of cancers at all ages were a result of occupation (Miller, 1984). It seems probable that the proportion of cancer resulting from occupational factors is decreasing in many developed countries, due to the introduction of appropriate control measures towards the end of the 20th century. The challenge for many developing countries, as they undertake the process of industrialization, is to ensure that they do not import the carcinogenic hazards related to various occupations.

One of the most common malignancies in sub-Saharan Africa and southeast Asia is cancer of the liver. The majority of these cases are a consequence of infection with hepatitis B virus or consumption of aflatoxin-contaminated

Cause of cancer (or contributory factor)	Best estimate	Range of acceptable estimates
Tobacco	30	25–40
Alcohol	3	2–4
Diet	35	10–70
Reproductive and sexual behaviour	7	1–13
Occupation	4	2–8
Pollution	2	1–5
Industrial by-products	1	1–2
Medicines and medical procedures	1	0.5–3
Geophysical factors	3	2–4
Infection	10	1–?

Table 2.1
Causes of Cancer Deaths in the United States of America (under age 65 years)

Source: Adapted from Doll R, Peto R. The causes of cancer: quantitative estimates of avoidable risks of cancer in the United States today. *Journal of the National Cancer Institute*, 1981, 66: 1191-1308

food (IARC, 1993, 1994b). In industrialized countries, primary liver cancer – though relatively uncommon – is mainly the result of excessive alcohol consumption (IARC, 1988).

The incidence of oesophageal and lung cancer and cancers of the colon and rectum, breast and prostate increases in parallel with economic development (Joint WHO/FAO expert consultation on diet, nutrition and the prevention of chronic diseases, in preparation). In developing countries, increased development is usually associated with many changes in diet and lifestyle. As a result, patterns of cancer tend to shift towards those of economically developed countries. Changes in lifestyle are also clearly associated with a greatly increased risk of ischaemic heart disease. This lifestyle is also clearly associated with a greatly increased risk of ischaemic heart disease. The risk of cancer can also be multiplied by risk factors acting simultaneously. For example, the effect of alcohol on oral, pharyngeal, laryngeal and oesophageal cancer risk is multiplied by the combined use of tobacco.

BURDEN OF CANCER

3

CANCER AS A WORLD HEALTH PROBLEM

Worldwide, there are over 10 million new cases of cancer and more than 6 million deaths from cancer annually. Two decades ago, these figures were 6 million and 4 million (Tomatis et al., 1990).

Of the 10 million new cancer cases each year, 4.7 million are in the more developed countries and nearly 5.5 million are in the less developed countries. Although the disease has often been regarded as a problem principally of the developed world, in fact, more than half of all cancers occur in the developing countries. In developed countries cancer is the second most common cause of death, and epidemiological evidence points to the emergence of a similar trend in developing countries. Cancer is currently the cause of 12% of all deaths worldwide (Table 3.1). In approximately 20 years time, the number of deaths annually due to cancer will increase from about 6 million to 10 million (see Table 3.2).

Table 3.1 Global and regional patterns of annual deaths, by cause, 2000

	Deaths from all causes (thousands)	Deaths from infectious & parasitic diseases (%)	Deaths from cancer (%)	Deaths from circulatory diseases (%)	Perinatal deaths (%)	Deaths from injury (%)	Deaths from other causes (%)
World total	55 694	25.9	12.6	30.0	4.4	9.1	18.0
More developed countries	13 594	6.0	21.6	47.9	0.7	7.9	15.9
Less developed countries	42 100	32.3	9.8	24.2	5.6	9.5	18.7
Africa	10 572	61.7	5.1	9.2	5.5	7.1	11.5
South and Central America	3 097	14.6	14.0	28.5	4.3	12.3	26.2
North America	2 778	6.3	23.8	41.0	0.6	6.4	21.9
Middle East	4 036	32.0	6.1	26.9	7.5	8.4	19.0
South-East Asia	14 157	29.9	8.0	28.9	7.1	9.7	16.4
Western Pacific	11 390	10.6	18.6	31.2	2.8	10.7	26.0
Europe	9 664	5.4	19.8	51.5	0.8	8.5	14.1

Source: WHO (2001c) *The World Health Report 2001.* WHO, Geneva

17

There are four principal reasons for the increase in cancer mortality:

- deaths from cardiovascular diseases are declining in developed countries;
- more people are surviving to old age, when cancer is more likely to occur;
- increasing tobacco use in recent decades has led to greater incidence of cancer of the lung and certain other sites;
- changes in diet, decreasing physical activity and increasing obesity have most likely contributed to an increase in various forms of cancer.

In developed countries, cancer generally accounts for about one-fifth of all deaths with mortality figures second only to those for cardiovascular diseases (see Table 3.1). Currently, infections and perinatal problems together account for less than 7% of the total mortality in developed countries, and the proportion is dropping. In these countries, of all major conditions that result in death, cancer is one of the very few for which the proportion is rising significantly (see Table 3.3).

In developing countries, cancer is now responsible for about one in 10 deaths (see Table 3.1), but incidence of the disease is increasing. As living standards improve and life expectancy is extended, the incidence of communicable diseases declines and noncommunicable diseases such as cancer assume greater importance.

CANCER OF VARIOUS SITES

Among men, lung and stomach cancer are the most common cancers worldwide, while prostate cancer is largely seen in more developed countries (see Table 3.4). For women, the most common cancers worldwide are breast and cervical cancer, although cervical cancer is primarily seen in less developed countries. Lung, colorectal and stomach cancer are among the five most common cancers for both men and women, in both more developed and less developed countries.

Further insights may be gained by considering the incidence of cancer of various parts of the body in different countries (see Table 3.5).

Table 3.2 Numbers of cancer deaths and new cancer cases in the world as estimated for 2000 and predicted for 2020[1]

Year	Region	New cases (millions)	Deaths (millions)
2000	More developed countries	4.7	2.6
	Less developed countries	5.4	3.6
	All countries	10.1	6.2
2020	More developed countries	6.0	3.5
	Less developed countries	9.3	6.3
	All countries	15.3	9.8

Source: Ferlay J. et al. *GLOBOCAN 2000: Cancer incidence, mortality and prevalence worldwide.* IARC
1 (based on population projections)

Table 3.3 Deaths from various major causes in selected countries, 1960, 1980 and 2000

	1960						1980						2000					
	Deaths from cancer (%)		Deaths from circulatory disease (%)		Deaths from other causes (%)		Deaths from cancer (%)		Deaths from circulatory disease (%)		Deaths from other causes (%)		Deaths from cancer (%)		Deaths from circulatory disease (%)		Deaths from other causes (%)	
	M	F	M	F	M	F	M	F	M	F	M	F	M	F	M	F	M	F
Australia	15	16	52	56	33	28	22	21	48	55	30	24	29	24	39	45	32	31
Chile	7	9	13	16	80	75	14	18	24	30	62	52	22	25	27	32	51	43
Japan	14	14	33	35	53	51	25	21	40	46	35	33	35	27	30	40	35	33
Portugal	9	10	26	33	65	57	16	14	39	47	45	39	25	20	40	53	35	27
Sweden	18	20	51	53	31	27	22	23	54	55	24	22	24	22	49	51	27	27
United Kingdom	20	18	49	56	31	26	24	21	49	51	27	28	27	23	42	43	31	34
USA	15	17	53	55	32	28	21	21	47	53	32	26	25	22	39	43	36	35

Sources: WHO (1963) Annual Epidemiological and Vital Statistics 1960 Geneva; WHO (1981) World Health Statistics Annual 1980–81 Geneva; WHO (2001c) The World Health Report 2001 Geneva

Table 3.4 Incidence of most common cancers, 2000

	Males			Females		
	Rank	Cancer	New cases (thousands)	Rank	Cancer	New cases (thousands)
World	1	Lung	902	1	Breast	1050
	2	Stomach	558	2	Cervix	471
	3	Prostate	543	3	Colon/rectum	446
	4	Colon/rectum	499	4	Lung	337
	5	Liver	398	5	Stomach	318
More developed countries	1	Lung	471	1	Breast	579
	2	Prostate	416	2	Colon/rectum	292
	3	Colon/rectum	319	3	Lung	175
	4	Stomach	208	4	Stomach	125
	5	Bladder	164	5	Corpus uteri	114
Less developed countries	1	Lung	431	1	Breast	471
	2	Stomach	350	2	Cervix	379
	3	Liver	325	3	Stomach	193
	4	Oesophagus	224	4	Lung	162
	5	Colon/rectum	180	5	Colon/rectum	154

Source: Ferlay J. et al. *GLOBOCAN 2000: Cancer incidence, mortality and prevalence worldwide.* IARC

Cancer of the oral cavity is particularly common in India and adjacent areas as a consequence of chewing tobacco. Stomach cancer is more common in China, Japan, and some countries of South and Central America and eastern Europe. Colorectal (large bowel) cancer is common in western societies, but has also become increasingly common in Japan. Liver cancer, though rare in most parts of the world, occurs more commonly in parts of Africa, eastern Asia, and the western Pacific. The incidence of lung cancer is high in North America and Europe and in Shanghai (China), but low in Africa. Epidemic levels of cigarette smoking account for the very high incidence of lung cancer in most of the developed countries, and recently this has become increasingly true of other parts of the world (Miller, 1999). Breast cancer, the commonest female cancer in the world, is very high in the West. Cervical cancer is more common in the developing than in the developed countries, and in many developing countries is the most frequent form of cancer in women. Prostate cancer is also common in the West. In the United States, the reported incidence of prostate cancer is extremely high, largely as a result of early detection through screening.

CANCER TRENDS OVER TIME

Ideally, a picture of a trend in a disease should be derived from data concerning incidence, that is, the number of new cases per population unit (usually

Table 3.5 Age-standardized cancer incidence: selected sites, selected registries, per 100 000, by sex

	Oral		Stomach		Colorectum		Liver		Lung		Breast	Cervix	Prostate
Registry	M	F	M	F	M	F	M	F	M	F	F	F	M
China (Shanghai)	1.0	0.8	46.5	21.0	21.5	18.1	28.2	9.8	56.1	18.2	26.5	3.3	2.3
Colombia (Cali)	2.3	1.4	33.3	19.3	11.9	10.8	2.6	2.2	24.4	9.5	38.8	34.4	32.7
England & Wales	1.5	0.7	16.1	6.3	33.9	23.7	2.0	1.0	62.4	22.8	68.8	12.5	28.0
India (Bombay)	6.2	4.6	7.7	3.8	7.6	5.6	3.9	1.9	14.5	3.7	28.2	20.2	7.9
Japan (Miyagi)	0.9	0.5	82.7	32.8	41.5	24.8	15.4	5.4	39.6	10.3	31.1	6.4	9.0
Uganda (Kyadondo)	1.0	1.7	5.4	3.2	7.5	5.1	9.9	4.7	4.2	0.4	20.7	40.8	27.7
Slovakia	5.4	0.4	24.5	10.3	40.6	23.6	7.2	3.1	79.1	8.7	38.6	16.4	22.0
USA, SEER (White)	3.0	1.6	7.5	3.1	42.4	29.5	3.0	1.2	61.3	33.8	90.7	7.5	100.8
USA, SEER (Black)	5.4	1.9	14.5	5.9	46.4	35.3	6.5	2.0	99.1	38.5	79.3	12.0	137.0

Source: Parkin DM et al. *Cancer incidence in five continents, Vol. VII,* Lyon, International Agency for Research on Cancer, 1997 (IARC Scientific Publications, No. 143).

100 000) per unit of time (usually per year). Unfortunately, such data can be obtained only from cancer registries or cancer surveys, both of which are relatively recent. Cancer mortality data, on the other hand, have been available for many countries during most of the 20th century, and can be used to study both geographical patterns and temporal changes in the disease.

Cancer deaths represent incidence indirectly, since they reflect the failure of treatment as well as the occurrence of the disease. For those forms of cancer for which available treatments are less effective, for example lung and stomach cancer, deaths reflect incidence quite accurately. Since 1950, the incidence of stomach cancer has declined by more than 50% in most countries. Lung cancer, by contrast, rose dramatically throughout the 20th century, more than 10-fold in North America for instance, although incidence in men began to decline in the 1980s, as it had earlier in the United Kingdom (Miller, 1999). Thus, cancer epidemics tend to rise to a peak and then recede over several decades. As a consequence, the time periods involved tend to conceal the epidemic nature of the trend.

Predictions of cancer prevalence, incidence, and mortality are important bases for cancer control activities. Together with predictions for other diseases, they are useful for setting national health priorities. As indicated in Chapter 1, major increases in cancer incidence and mortality are predicted for the developing countries.

PSYCHOSOCIAL AND ECONOMIC IMPACTS OF CANCER

Regardless of prognosis, the initial diagnosis of cancer is still perceived by many patients as a life-threatening event. Over one-third of patients experience clinical range anxiety and/or depression (Epping-Jordan, 1999). Surprisingly, disease severity, prognosis, and type of treatment do not seem to have a large impact on psychosocial adjustment to cancer. However, patients who can find a sense of meaning in what is happening to them and who can achieve mastery over their illness adjust well to their cancer.

Cancer can be equally, if not more, distressing for family and friends. Family income loss, social isolation, family tensions, and adverse effects on daily functioning in the family may follow closely on the occurrence of cancer. Similarly, health care providers are not immune to the psychosocial effects of caring for people with cancer. Workers who frequently see sick and dying patients, or who cannot provide assistance to their patients in the manner they want, are at risk for "staff burn-out". This syndrome is characterized by emotional exhaustion and de-personalization of the patient, and has been linked to job absenteeism, insomnia, substance abuse and physical complaints (Ullrich, Fitzgerald, 1990).

21

The economic burden of cancer is most obvious in health care costs, such as those for hospitals, other health services, and drugs. Indirect costs arise from loss of productivity as a result of the illness and premature death of those affected. Direct costs may be estimated fairly readily in situations where the nature and extent of services provided to cancer patients are known. Calculation of indirect costs, however, involves making assumptions concerning both expected future earnings and a discount rate to convert potential earnings into a current amount. One estimate of direct cancer care costs in the United States of America in 1990 was US$ 27.5 billion, the corresponding indirect costs of premature mortality from cancer amounting to almost US$ 59 billion (Brown, Hodgson, Rice, 1996).

Beyond these numbers, the common reality, especially in poor areas, is a profound economic family crisis. A diagnosis of cancer in one of the adults in a family may lead not only to the loss of a source of income, but also all too frequently to exhausting the family's remaining income and resources in seeking treatments. Perhaps saddest of all are the futile frantic searches and large amounts of money paid by the family for treatments that cannot prolong the life of the family member with advanced cancer. If families feel abandoned by their formal health care system, they may spend their remaining resources seeking assistance from well-meaning or unscrupulous individuals who falsely promise to help.

Approaches to Cancer Control

The four principal approaches to cancer control are:

Prevention Prevention means eliminating or minimizing exposure to the causes of cancer, and includes reducing individual susceptibility to the effect of such causes. This approach offers the greatest public health potential and the most cost-effective long-term method of cancer control. Tobacco is the leading single cause of cancer worldwide and in the fight against cancer every country should give highest priority to tobacco control.

Early detection Increasing awareness of the signs and symptoms of cancer contributes to early detection of the disease. Where tests for cancer of specific sites are available, and facilities are appropriate, screening of apparently healthy individuals can disclose cancer in early or precursor stages, when treatment may be most effective. Early detection is only successful when linked to effective treatment.

Diagnosis and treatment Cancer diagnosis calls for a combination of careful clinical assessment and diagnostic investigations. Once a diagnosis is confirmed, it is necessary to ascertain cancer staging to evaluate the extension of the disease and be able to provide treatment accordingly. Cancer treatment aims at curing, prolonging useful life and improving quality of life. Treatment services should give priority to early detectable tumours and potentially curable cancers. In addition, treatment approaches should include psychosocial support, rehabilitation and close coordination with palliative care to ensure the best possible quality of life for cancer patients.

Palliative care In most of the world, the majority of the cancer patients present with advanced disease. For them, the only realistic treatment option is pain relief and palliative care. Effective approaches to palliative care are available to improve the quality of life for cancer patients.

The scientific basis for these approaches to cancer control is considered in Chapters 4–7 of this monograph. Cancer control research is briefly discussed in Chapter 8, while Chapter 9 reviews cancer surveillance, the basis for cancer control planning, monitoring and evaluation.

PART

II

PREVENTION

4

Cancer prevention should be a key element in all national cancer control programmes. Prevention not only focuses on the risks associated with a particular illness or problem but also on protective factors. Among prevention activities, emphasis should be placed on:

– tobacco control;
– healthy diet;
– physical activities and avoidance of obesity;
– reducing alcohol use;
– reducing carcinogenic occupational and environmental exposures;
– immunization against hepatitis B virus;
– combating schistosomiasis;
– avoidance of prolonged exposure to the sun;
– health education, relating to sexual and reproductive factors associated with cancer.

Action on tobacco use is universally needed, but the priorities accorded to other components of the programme will depend on the results of a situation analysis of the country concerned, covering the actual and forecast burden of cancer cases in the country, and the estimated proportion of potentially preventable cases. A broad range of health promotion activities are appropriate to cancer control and these are examined in detail at the end of this chapter.

TOBACCO

Tobacco dependence

Tobacco dependence is listed in the WHO ICD-10 as a chronic condition in the section on mental and behavioural disorders (WHO, 1992). Such dependence syndromes are described as a cluster of behavioural, cognitive and physiological phenomena that develop after repeated substance use and that typically include a strong desire to take the drug, difficulties in controlling its use and persistence in drug use despite harmful consequences.

The use of tobacco in any of its several forms has extended over much of the world. Young people usually encounter the practice among their peers, and may then take up the habit themselves. Typically, tobacco use begins through social contacts, but the habit is reinforced by the development of physiological dependence, derived from the nicotine content of tobacco. Cessation of tobacco use in those who are addicted produces withdrawal symptoms, typical of other addictions. Such symptoms can appear within hours of cessation and persist for weeks or months.

Tobacco is smoked, chewed and dipped in various forms around the world. Tobacco is also consumed frequently as a mixture with other substances. On the Indian subcontinent and adjacent parts of central Asia, for example, tobacco is often mixed in a quid with betel nut and lime, and retained in the mouth for long periods of time. In Sudan, the use of smokeless tobacco in the form of snuff, called toombak, is widespread. Toombak is dipped in the saliva of the oral cavity or, less frequently, sniffed into the nasal cavities. Today, in most parts of the world, cigarette smoking is the most common form of tobacco use.

Health significance of tobacco use

Although the adverse health consequences of tobacco use have been recognized for over 50 years, it is the major epidemiological studies that revealed the full extent of tobacco-related health damage (IARC, 1986).

Lung cancer was rare in North America and Europe during the early 20th century, but its incidence began to increase substantially about 15 years after the First World War, in the wake of heavy smoking among members of the armed forces. A similar increase in the incidence among women was noted in the 1960s, following 15–20 years of cigarette consumption that started during the Second World War. During the period 1950–2000, smoking accounted for 50 million deaths in males and 10 million in females in developed countries (Peto et al., 1994). Now, the epidemic is extending into many developing countries, where smoking has been encouraged by the marketing policies of national and multinational tobacco companies.

In industrialized countries, 80–90% of lung cancers are attributable to tobacco smoking. The longer a person has been smoking and the more packs per day smoked, the greater the risk. If a person stops smoking before a cancer develops, the risk remains at the same level or may even increase. Even after ten years, the ex-smoker's risk still does not equal the lower risk of a person who never took up smoking. Cigar smoking and pipe smoking are almost as likely to cause lung cancer as cigarette smoking.

A substantial proportion of cancer in the oral cavity, pharynx, larynx, pancreas, kidney, oesophagus, bladder, and probably stomach and cervix uteri is also attributable to tobacco. Moreover, smoking is responsible for a large amount of chronic lung disease and contributes heavily to cardio-vascular disease. Tobacco smoke contains approximately 4000 chemical substances, of which at least 438 can produce cancer. The most dangerous are nicotine, tobacco tar, and carbon monoxide. The most common cancer causing agents in tobacco are the polyaromatic hydrocarbon and nitroso compounds. The development of cancer in particular organs depends upon the sites that come into contact with the chemical constituents of tobacco and tobacco smoke. The lungs are the principal target when tobacco smoke is inhaled; when tobacco is chewed or kept in the mouth, the cheek, tongue, and other parts of the oral cavity are affected. The increased risk at other sites is probably a result of carcinogens being absorbed into the blood-stream from the lungs and transported to the relevant organ.

One critical aspect of tobacco relevant to cancer control is the effect of passive exposure to smoke in increasing the risk of cancer of the lung and possibly of other sites in non-smokers (IARC, 1986). Non-smokers who breathe in the smoke of others (also called second-hand smoke or environ-mental tobacco smoke) are at increased risk for lung cancer. A non-smoker who is married to a smoker has a 20–30% greater risk of developing lung cancer than the non-smoking spouse of a non-smoker. Workers who have been exposed to tobacco smoke in the workplace are also more likely to get lung cancer.

Action against tobacco

The need for effective global action against the tobacco epidemic is urgent, especially in developing countries. Hundreds of millions of people cur-rently use tobacco, and tens of millions will suffer severely impaired health and shortened lives. Effective tobacco control begins with the realization that tobacco is powerfully addictive. The task of containing the spread of tobacco use and assisting individuals to overcome the addiction may be achieved in a number of ways, but must always take account of the wide-spread, longstanding, and deeply ingrained nature of the habit and the strong social factors that encourage it, as well as the political imperatives of many countries, especially those with a major indigenous tobacco industry.

Many countries have undertaken health promotion and health education programmes to inform people of the adverse effects of tobacco. However, these efforts are continually undermined by the tobacco industry (WHO, 1998c). Decades of experience demonstrate that health promotion and edu-cation measures are insufficient to combat the tobacco problem. For more effective results, health promotion and education must be accompanied by other actions, particularly legislation, tobacco taxes and tobacco cessation programmes, that will reduce the social acceptability of tobacco use. Much depends on people having adequate understanding of both the short-term and long-term consequences of the habit, but simply imparting this knowledge is not enough. Equally important is the cultivation of attitudes that will be effective against smoking or other use of tobacco. These attitudes may reflect personal values regarding short-term effects (on personal appearance, for instance) as much as concern about long-term health damage. Young people are sensitive to the way in which tobacco remnants and the odour of smoke on their person and their clothes may affect their social relationships. In addition, they need psychosocial resistance skills, particularly in situations where there is substantial pressure to initiate or continue tobacco use. Education techniques have been developed to help in these situations. Teaching social resistance skills in school can do much to help youngsters aged 10–15 years to avoid cigarette smoking.

Overall, direct efforts to influence the behaviour of the individual with regard to tobacco have had, and will probably continue to have, only limited success. Mass education, however, and development of public attitudes against tobacco use have encouraged many cigarette smokers to give up the habit. In North America, where cigarette smoking is in decline, most people who have given up cigarettes report that they did so "on their own"; they took personal responsibility for their action. People with higher levels of education and greater concern about health, especially physicians and other health professionals, tend to be the first to give up smoking. In developing countries, the first people to become relatively affluent – and therefore to have the money for cigarettes – are also the first to start smoking. As they acquire knowledge of the threat to health, they are also the first to give up the habit. This diffusion of the tobacco epidemic extends throughout society, until it is the least well educated, and most socially disadvantaged segments of society that retain the habit, and the consequences to their health. The trend to resist smoking can also be accelerated by specific counselling and advice from physicians. Professional health workers should be influenced by the policies of the health services in which they work; they should avoid tobacco use of any sort in order to set an example to others.

Government action can do much to encourage people to give up cigarettes, by prohibiting smoking in workplaces, restaurants, and public buildings, and on public transport, for example, and by controlling the advertising of tobacco products, providing the regulations are enforced. Valuable use can be made of the media for mass education about the dangers of smoking and means of avoiding or overcoming the habit. In communities where smoking has become socially unacceptable and non-smokers are in the majority, there are major incentives not to smoke.

Government economic policy towards tobacco is highly relevant to individual and mass education against tobacco use. The powerful commercial interests involved in production and distribution of tobacco products exploit people's dependence on tobacco in order to maintain sales. Their arguments include the preservation of "free" trade and of individual "freedom" to enjoy tobacco, as well as the need to avoid economic problems in the form of loss of jobs and material investment in the tobacco industry. Strong political and social initiatives to counteract these pressures are vital. Government action regarding land use, subsidies, taxes, and other leverage on prices also has a profound influence on the spread of tobacco use. The stringency of measures taken by some countries to prevent use of other dependence-producing substances contrasts with their policies on tobacco, yet tobacco is responsible for far more deaths than heroin and cocaine combined. A number of countries impose severe penalties on those involved in the illicit drug trade, yet continue to subsidize the tobacco industry. Increasing the price of tobacco products by taxation can help to reduce tobacco use, especially among young people and others whose purchases are strongly influenced by price. Elimination of tobacco prices as an element of the cost-of-living index in various countries would also be beneficial.

As national policies against tobacco use are established and implemented, it becomes important to guard against attempts by the tobacco industry to switch its manufacturing emphasis to products other than cigarettes. Snuff is an example of such a product, with sales primarily aimed at boys aged 10–15 years. The objective is seemingly to encourage dependence among young people on alternative tobacco products which pose less well-known threats to health and are, as yet, less deprecated than cigarettes. It is, therefore, essential to educate people about the dangers of such products, by means such as explicit warning labels on packages.

International aspects

International collaboration over taxation policies is essential, because international expansion is as much an objective of the tobacco industry as of any other industry. Heavy and unchecked pressure by multinational tobacco companies is helping to spread the habit of cigarette smoking in the developing countries. Around 1990, eight of the ten countries with the highest smoking rates among males (70–95%) were in the developing world, and included about one-quarter of the world's population. At that time the smoking prevalence rate for males was estimated to be 51% in developed countries and 54% in developing countries. The corresponding estimates for females were 21% and 8% (Stanley, 1993).

Companies based in the most technically advanced countries seek to expand both their markets and their opportunities for investment in tobacco production. This is particularly true where home markets are declining in the face of public opinion and government legislation on smoking. International companies seek links with companies in the target countries as a means of strengthening political commitment to the tobacco industry in those countries. Such tendencies should be resisted where possible. Countries have a responsibility to avoid exporting carcinogens, in whatever form, to any other country, especially to less advantaged nations. The World Bank has exercised important leadership in refusing loans to countries for tobacco projects. In 1998, the Secretary-General of the United Nations designated an ad hoc Inter-Agency Task Force on Tobacco Control, under the leadership of WHO, to galvanize global support for tobacco control. Since the inception of the Task Force, new inter-agency partnerships have been initiated in several areas, including close collaboration between WHO, The World Bank, FAO and ILO on the economics of tobacco control, and supply and production issues.

Success in controlling tobacco use

Efforts to achieve control of tobacco have met with some success. Political will to tackle the issue is a paramount consideration and has been expressed in legislative action of various sorts by more than 70 countries. WHO is working to reinforce and strengthen national legislative processes by promoting an International Framework Convention for Tobacco Control (FCTC). In 1999, the World Health Assembly, comprising the 191 WHO Member States, adopted resolution WHA 52.18 initiating the development of the Framework Convention.

The FCTC holds the potential for advancing global cooperation for tobacco control. The principles, norms and standards laid down in the Convention establish priorities for national legislative action and multilateral cooperation for tobacco control. According to treaty law and practice, the FCTC standards will form the minimum content of national tobacco control legislation within parties, subject to any reservations under the treaty. This is without prejudice to stronger national legislation that countries may enact. Treaty institutions established under the Convention could stimulate financial, technical and other assistance programmes for national tobacco control legislation. By providing a multilateral and institutionalized forum for consultations on tobacco control, the FCTC will promote the adoption and implementation of effective tobacco control legislation and other strategies worldwide. The legislation is intended to:

- Set out government policy on the production, promotion, and use of tobacco;
- Encourage those who already smoke to stop, and dissuade others, particu-

larly young people, from starting;

- Protect the right of non-smokers to be free from passive smoking and to breathe clean air;
- Contribute to the development of a social climate in which smoking is unacceptable;
- Provide a rational basis for the allocation of resources to effective anti-smoking programmes;
- Control smuggling of tobacco products.

Education programmes directed against smoking must be complemented by legislation. In Sweden, for example, strong health warnings on tobacco became mandatory in 1975, and the number of daily smokers fell from 43% of the population in 1976 to 31% in 1980. The decline was especially pronounced among teenagers, apparently in response to the compulsory education about smoking and health in schools. The remarkably high price elasticity of demand for tobacco products may be seen in the substantial decrease in cigarette consumption among teenagers that follows a price increase. Successive tax increases in South Africa resulted in substantial reductions in cigarette sales, and consumption in Canada declined markedly in response to increases in taxes in the 1980s, until perturbed by a reduction in tobacco taxes in an attempt to reduce smuggling of tobacco from the United States. In 1983, France began to levy a tax on alcohol and tobacco; proceeds go to the National Health Insurance Fund to help offset the extra health care costs resulting from the use of those substances. Countries such as Australia, Egypt, the Islamic Republic of Iran, and Thailand, and several US states, including California and Massachusetts, earmark a portion of tobacco taxes to fund tobacco control programme activities such as counter-advertising or broader public health activities.

The total impact of campaigns in various countries is already substantial. In the United States of America, the 1964 report of the Surgeon-General (US Department of Health, Education and Welfare, 1964) resulted in a campaign against cigarettes which led to a drop in cigarette smoking from 45% of the adult population to 30% two decades later, and the decline continued thereafter.

The most favourable results have been seen in countries that have implemented comprehensive tobacco control policies and programmes that ban advertising, place strong warnings on packages, implement controls on the use of tobacco in public places, levy high taxes on tobacco, and provide effective education and cessation programmes. From 1970 to 1995, comprehensive tobacco control policies were implemented, maintained and upgraded in Australia, Finland, France, Iceland, New Zealand, Norway, Portugal, Singapore, Sweden and Thailand. Tobacco consumption has remained low or is falling rapidly in these countries, providing clear evidence that the more comprehensive the policy, the more effective the solution. In other countries, partial tobacco control policies and programmes have produced only partial solutions.

A national cancer control programme is an ideal vehicle for tobacco control activities which, if undertaken in isolation, might be rejected for political reasons by ministries of finance and agriculture. Effective tobacco control activities will reduce the incidence of smoking-associated cancers, and also of other conditions for which tobacco is a risk factor, such as cardiovascular disease, respiratory disease, and perinatal mortality. The effect of passive smoking on the incidence of respiratory disease in infants and children, and of lung cancer and probably other cancers in non-smokers shows that tobacco use is not purely a personal responsibility. Serious commitment by the responsible authorities in each country is essential if effective measures to reduce tobacco use are to be implemented. Relevant decisions will have to be taken at the highest level of government to avoid any potential conflict between policies adopted by different ministries.

In developing tobacco control programmes, both general and specific objectives should be formulated. The general objective should take account of the fact that in developed countries about one-third of all cancers are tobacco-related, and thus might be stated as follows: *to reduce the incidence of the cancers caused by tobacco.*

More specific objectives may include the following:
- to reduce the number of young people starting smoking;
- to increase the number of people giving up smoking;
- to educate all schoolchildren about the effects of tobacco on health;
- to inform everyone in the population, smokers and non-smokers, of the risks of smoking;
- to inform smokers about the benefits of giving up smoking and how they can do so;
- to provide support and assistance to people who want to stop smoking;
- to create a smoke-free environment.

These objectives should be supplemented with a set of specific targets or quantitative goals that will enable progress to be assessed in the future. Targets will vary from country to country depending on the prevalence of smoking, but a typical target for the first specific objective might be:
- the proportion of young people who are regular cigarette smokers will be reduced from the 2002 level of x% to y% by the year 2012.

It is important to set realistic targets: failure to achieve them could have adverse effects on public acceptance of the national cancer control programme as a whole.

Processes need to be set out to achieve the objectives of the programme. They may be relatively inexpensive to implement, but their effects are substantial. They include:

- establishing clear policy on legislative measures, particularly price increases and taxation on cigarettes;
- establishing a national, multidisciplinary tobacco control committee, with members drawn from all concerned government ministries and from non-governmental organizations that can advise on strategies appropriate to the national culture;
- developing human, financial and structural resources with long-term sustainability to support tobacco control;
- establishing a national focal point to stimulate, support and coordinate activities;
- establishing effective programmes of education and public information on tobacco and health, including smoking cessation programmes, with active involvement of health professionals and the media.

Evaluation of the programme's success in achieving expected outcomes requires the following:

- In the short term, a prevalence study of tobacco use to determine the proportion of adolescents and adults who regularly smoke or chew tobacco, as well as information from such a survey or from other data on:
  - the percentage of school curricula and adult literacy programmes that include information on tobacco;
  - the percentage of health professional education programmes and continuing education programmes that include information on tobacco.
- In the medium term, assessment of changes in the incidence of tobacco-associated conditions other than cancer, such as coronary heart disease, and cardiovascular and respiratory diseases.
- In the long term, assessment of the reduction in mortality resulting from lung cancer and other tobacco-linked cancers, and in chronic obstructive lung disease.

Sample sizes for prevalence studies should be sufficiently large to allow the monitoring of changes in risk groups, for example, male/female, urban/rural, young/old, high/low socioeconomic group. Such studies should be undertaken during implementation of the programme and at regular intervals thereafter.

DIET

Some patterns of food intake may be causally related to cancer while others may protect against the disease (World Cancer Research Fund, American Institute for Cancer Research, 1997; Key et al., in preparation). Evidence for a quantitative relationship between cancer and food or specific nutrients is, however, not as strong as the evidence for the relationship between cancer and tobacco, or alcohol, or some chemical exposures. Nevertheless, it is thought that dietary factors may be associated with about 30% of cancers in developed countries and perhaps 20% of cancers in developing countries (Key et al., in preparation). Therefore, serious consideration should be given to dietary modification as a means of preventing the disease. A summary of the most recent evidence on the relationship between diet and cancer is given in Table 4.1 (Joint WHO/FAO expert consultation on diet, nutrition and the prevention of chronic diseases, in preparation).

Fruits and vegetables

The incidence of a number of cancers is low in populations that consume substantial quantities of plant foods, especially of vegetables and fruit (World Cancer Research Fund, American Institute for Cancer Research, 1997). For colorectal cancer, the evidence for a protective effect of fruit and vegetable intake is relatively strong. For other cancers, evidence for a protective effect of some constituents of fruits or vegetables is growing, although for many of the cancer types the available data may only have permitted the analysis of a factor that should be regarded as an index of consumption of plant foods.

Table 4.1 Diet, physical activity and cancer: levels of evidence based on a recent review

Level of evidence	Decrease risk	Increase risk
Convincing	Physical activity[1]	Overweight and obesity[2] Alcohol[3] Chinese-style salted fish[4] Some mycotoxins (aflatoxin)[5]
Probable	Fruit and vegetables[6] Physical activity[8]	Preserved meat and red meat[1] Salt preserved foods & salt[7] Very hot food and drinks[9]
Insufficient	Fibre, soya, fish, n-3 fatty acids, carotenoids, vitamins B_2, B_6, folate, B_{12}, C, D, E, calcium, zinc, selenium, non-nutrient plant constituents	Animal fats, heterocyclic amines, polycyclic aromatic hydrocarbons, nitrosamines

Source: Joint WHO/FAO expert consultation on diet, nutrition and the prevention of chronic diseases, in preparation

1. Colorectum
2. Oesophagus, colorectum, breast, endometrium, kidney
3. Oral cavity, pharynx, larynx, oesophagus, liver, breast
4. Nasopharynx
5. Liver
6. Oral cavity, oesophagus, stomach, colorectum
7. Stomach
8. Breast
9. Oral cavity, pharynx, oesophagus

For breast cancer, recent analyses of cohort studies have produced inconsistent results. Several studies on stomach cancer have produced consistent evidence of a protective effect of vitamin C. As discussed below, this is likely to reflect the efficacy of this vitamin in inhibiting nitrosamine production (Tomatis et al., 1990).

Protective effects against lung cancer were ascribed to betacarotene, although indices of consumption of betacarotene are largely derived from estimated intake of various vegetables. However, in trials of betacarotene as a chemopreventive agent in heavy smokers and asbestos workers, higher risks of lung cancer were seen in those receiving betacarotene than in the controls (The Alpha-Tocopharol, Beta Carotene Cancer Prevention Study Group, 1994; Omenn et al., 1996). IARC has concluded that betacarotene should not be used as a dietary supplement in humans (IARC, 1998a). It has also concluded that there is no good evidence that vitamin A *per se* is protective (IARC, 1998b).

Protective effects of fruit and vegetable consumption probably extend to oral, oesophageal and stomach cancers (Key et al., in preparation).

Dietary fat

International comparisons indicate a high correlation between dietary fat intake and the occurrence of cancer of the breast, prostate, uterus (body), ovary, and colon. These data parallel the results of animal experiments, as well as a number of epidemiological studies, though recently some cohort studies have failed to confirm the associations noted in previous case-control studies, especially for breast cancer (Hunter et al., 1996), thus casting doubt on the causal nature of the associations. Part of the difficulty could be in accurate quantification of dietary fat consumption at the relevant time in the natural history of many cancers, so that cohort studies may simply be failing to find an association due to a lack of precision in the measurement. In animal studies, polyunsaturated fat appears to increase risk; however the epidemiological studies do not support that in humans.

Meat

There is some evidence that consumption of red meat and, perhaps in particular processed meat, increases the risk of colon cancer (Key et al in preparation). Whether this is a direct effect of substances in red meat, such as saturated fat, or the effect of cooking or food processing methods is uncertain. In nearly every cancer site for which the effect of white meat (for example, chicken) or fish consumption has been evaluated, no increase in risk has been found.

35

Nitrites and salt

Studies of the declining incidence of stomach cancer have suggested that this trend is related to changes in dietary patterns, particularly the decrease in salting and pickling for food preservation, the increasing use of refrigeration and the associated increase in the availability of fruits and vegetables (and thus vitamin C) year round. Salting and pickling involve certain chemicals that are known to combine with amines in the stomach to produce nitrosamines—powerful carcinogenic agents. This mechanism may account for the high incidence of stomach cancer in some areas of Japan and certain other parts of the world, such as Chile and Costa Rica; the hypothesis is supported by epidemiological studies in North America and Europe (World Cancer Research Fund, American Institute for Cancer Research, 1997). Nasopharyngeal cancer, common in South Asia, has been consistently associated with a high intake of Chinese-style salted fish, a special product which is usually softened by partial decomposition before or during salting (Key et al in preparation).

Further prospective data are needed, in particular to examine whether some of the dietary associations may be partly confounded by *Helicobacter pylori* infection and whether dietary factors may modify the association of *Helicobacter pylori* with risk.

Contaminants

Certain substances naturally present in food and other substances generated during its preparation have carcinogenic potential. Additionally, food may become contaminated with chemicals capable of causing cancer. In Africa and some parts of Asia, for instance, the growth of mould on nuts and other foods under particular conditions of storage produces aflatoxin, a highly potent carcinogen strongly implicated in the high incidence of liver cancer (IARC, 1993). Generally, however, food contaminants are responsible for only a small amount of diet-induced cancer (Tomatis et al., 1990).

Additives

Substances added to food as preservatives or to enhance colour may also be carcinogenic. Since 1956, the Food and Agriculture Organization/World Health Organization (FAO/WHO) Food Standards Programme has set maximum levels for additives, contaminants, and pesticide residues to minimize this possibility. These standards are implemented by the Codex Alimentarius Commission. It seems unlikely that currently permitted additives have any significant effect in increasing the risk of cancer (Tomatis et al., 1990).

Promoting dietary modification

Prevention of cancer by dietary means can be encouraged by observing the following public health goal (World Cancer Research Fund, American Institute for Cancer Research, 1997; Joint WHO/FAO expert consultation on diet, nutrition and the prevention of chronic diseases, in preparation): populations should consume nutritionally adequate and varied diets, based primarily on foods of plant origin.

In addition, the following measures should be advocated for individuals:

1. Maintain body mass index (BMI) in range of 18.5 to 25 kg/m^2, and avoid weight gain in adulthood.
2. Engage in regular physical activity.
3. Consumption of alcoholic beverages is not recommended: if consumed, do not exceed 2 units per day (1 unit is equivalent to approximately 10 g of alcohol and is provided by one glass of beer, wine or spirits).
4. Minimize exposure to aflatoxin in foods.
5. Chinese-style salted fish should only be eaten in moderation, especially during childhood. Overall consumption of salt-preserved foods and salt should be moderate.
6. Have a diet which includes at least 400 g/day of fruit and vegetables.
7. Meat: those who are not vegetarian are advised to moderate consumption of preserved meat (e.g. sausages, salami, bacon, ham etc.) and red meat (e.g. beef, pork, lamb). Poultry and fish (except Chinese-style salted fish, see 5. above) have been studied and found not to be associated with increased cancer risk.
8. Do not consume very hot foods or drinks.

Countries in which the traditional diet results in a low incidence of diet-associated cancers should take action to ensure that their patterns of food consumption do not change to those of North America and western Europe.

A national cancer control programme offers an opportunity to implement the recommendations of the WHO Study Group on diet, nutrition, and the prevention of chronic disease (WHO, 1990a), the World Cancer Research Fund and American Institute for Cancer Research (1997), and the recent WHO/FAO expert consultation (Joint WHO/FAO expert consultation on diet, nutrition and the prevention of chronic diseases, in preparation).

Among the measures to be considered to promote dietary modification are the following:

• government recognition of dietary factors in cancer etiology and consideration of the implications of those factors for the relevant ministries

(especially health and agriculture);
- appropriate education on diet in schools;
- public education campaigns about diet for adults;
- collaboration with representatives of the food industry (both production and service sectors) to ensure compliance with the nutritional objectives of the programme.

An international strategy comparable to that currently underway for tobacco can be envisaged.

ALCOHOL

Health significance of alcohol

Besides the toxicity of excessive alcohol intake, and the tendency for some individuals to become dependent on alcohol, investigation has also disclosed long-term damage caused by alcohol to the nervous system, the liver, and other organs. These effects often result from years of exposure, generally to levels lower than either those that cause gross intoxication or that are consumed by those with alcohol dependence.

The consumption of alcoholic beverages convincingly increases the risk of cancers of the oral cavity, pharynx, larynx, oesophagus, liver, and breast (and probably colorectum). The increase in risk appears to be primarily due to alcohol *per se* rather than specific alcoholic beverages. Whereas most of the excess risks occur with high alcohol consumption, a small (about 10%) increase in risk of breast cancer has been observed with approximately one drink per day. Recent studies suggest that the excess risk of breast and colon cancer associated with alcohol consumption may be concentrated in persons with low folate intake (Key et al., in preparation).

The carcinogenic effect of alcohol in relation to oral, pharyngeal, laryngeal and oesophageal cancer is exacerbated by tobacco use (IARC, 1988). Primary liver cancer is strongly associated with cirrhosis of the liver, whether induced by toxic or infectious agents. In developed countries, cirrhosis is related principally to alcohol consumption.

The risk relationship between alcohol and cancer is nearly a linear dose-response relationship between volume of drinking and risk. The pattern of drinking does not seem to have an important role. There is little evidence to suggest that consumption of small amounts of alcohol increases the risk of cancer. Moreover, there is evidence that moderate alcohol consumption (no more than two drinks in a single day) is protective for cardiovascular disease.

These patterns are substantially different from the risks of tobacco smoking,
where any degree of exposure, active or passive, is hazardous.

Controlling alcohol consumption

In any approach to the control of alcohol consumption, it is useful to note several similarities with the problem of tobacco. Both substances are:
- toxic agents that can damage several parts of the body, and also cause cancer;
- favoured by economic advance in developing countries, or among disadvantaged people in developed countries;
- widely supported by social forces such as peer pressure;
- likely to produce or capable of producing physiological dependence;
- backed by strong commercial interests;
- "price elastic", that is, consumption goes down as their cost to the individual goes up.

Control of alcohol must take into account the wide range of social forces that affect alcohol use. In many Muslim countries, the sale and consumption of alcohol are prohibited whereas in many other countries, wine at mealtimes is the social norm and certain groups are especially heavy consumers of stronger alcoholic beverages. Efforts to control alcohol will usually reflect concern about a range of diseases, as well as the domestic, social, and industrial problems that arise from alcohol use. Hence, specific action against alcohol will rarely be justified solely as part of a national cancer control programme. Those involved in cancer control must collaborate with other health interests in seeking to reduce excessive alcohol use and to provide public education about the effects of alcohol on health.

Reducing individual consumption is potentially a powerful strategy against alcohol abuse. However, action directed solely to individuals (in the form of brief interview sessions or alcohol dependence treatment) is unlikely to be fully effective. Practical obstacles to the use of alcohol are required. The most effective action a government can take to reduce individual alcohol consumption is to raise prices through taxation. Other measures that have been tried with varying degrees of success include limiting the places and times at which alcohol is available, raising the age at which alcohol may be purchased, and creating a government monopoly on alcohol sales.

Health promotion activities to reduce alcohol consumption consist of taxation, general public education, and encouraging highly vulnerable groups, such as young people, to avoid or significantly reduce consumption of alcoholic beverages by providing early interventions for those drinking at hazardous levels. Programmes targeting particularly hazardous situations, such as drinking alcohol and driving, may also be effective. It is important to identify individuals who show signs of alcohol dependence and to provide help. This help can come from health professionals or from self-help groups.

Physical activity and avoidance of obesity

Obesity is epidemic in many developed countries, and is increasingly becoming a concern in many developing countries. Obesity is defined by WHO as a body mass index (BMI) of $\geq 30\,kg/m^2$, while people with BMI in the range $\geq 25 - <30\,kg/m^2$ are classified as overweight. The prevalence of obesity in the Unites States of America has increased to about 22% of adults, with another 32% of adults being classified as overweight. In Europe, about half the adult population is overweight, and the prevalence of obesity in the urban areas of many developing countries is similar.

Obesity increases the risk of postmenopausal breast cancer, and cancers of the endometrium, colorectum, kidney, and oesophagus. It is also associated with cardiovascular disease and adult-onset diabetes. The fundamental causes of obesity and overweight are societal, resulting from an environment that promotes sedentary lifestyles and over-consumption of high-calorific food. There is also convincing evidence to show that physical activity has a beneficial influence on the risk of colorectal cancer and probably has a beneficial effect on breast cancer risk, independent of its effect on obesity. Taken together, excess body weight and physical inactivity account for approximately one-quarter to one-third of breast cancer, and cancers of the colon, endometrium, kidney (renal cell) and oesophagus (adenocarcinoma).

Moderate activities, such as walking for one hour a day is required to maintain normal body weight, especially in sedentary people. In addition, more vigorous activities such as brisk walking several times a week may give additional benefit concerning cancer prevention. However, obesity cannot be prevented or managed, nor physical activity promoted, solely at the level of the individual. Governments, the food industry, the media, communities and individuals all need to work together to modify the environment so that it is less conducive to weight gain (IARC, 2001). In developing countries without a current obesity problem, the objective should be to enact strategies to prevent their situation from worsening.

As countries industrialize, and the size of their agrarian sector is reduced, a higher proportion of the population has lowered energy expenditure. Sedentary jobs replace more active occupations. As populations become more urbanized, mechanical transportation replaces walking or bicycling, and another source of energy expenditure is reduced. Some modern urban designs make pedestrian activity unsafe, and a substantial distance between residential areas and workplaces or markets makes using a motor vehicle virtually inevitable. Prevention of the epidemic of obesity and inactivity characteristic of many developed countries is an important part of cancer prevention strategies, in addition to having beneficial effects on cardiovascular disease and diabetes risks.

OCCUPATION AND ENVIRONMENT

It appears that occupational factors are responsible for about 5–10% of all cancers and that environmental factors are responsible for 1–2% of all cancers in industrialized countries. While it is essential to minimize occupational and environmental exposure to carcinogens, the level of public concern may well be disproportionate to the dangers.

Knowledge about occupation and cancer

Historically, exposure of chimney sweeps to soot and of other workers to certain types of mineral oil were found to cause cancer of the scrotum; metal mining gave rise to lung cancer, and chemicals used in dye works to bladder cancer (Tomatis et al., 1990). Systematic investigations have disclosed many more such links throughout the industrialized world. Moreover, the expansion of many industries has accelerated the introduction of new physical and chemical processes that entail exposure to carcinogenic agents.

Identification of occupational factors in cancer etiology is hindered by the fact that as many as 20–30 years may elapse between exposure and disease. However, the concentration of exposure among relatively few workers has made it possible to pinpoint several occupational situations responsible for a variety of cancers. Some examples of the occupations involved are given in Table 4.2.

In industrialized countries, approximately 9% of all malignancies among men result from exposure to carcinogens in the workplace (Miller, 1984); the figure is lower for women. In different regions there may be substantial differences in the amount of cancer attributable to occupation, dependent on the prevailing industries in the area (Vineis et al., 1988). Risk is generally apparent from the age of about 50 years, but maximum risk may not be seen until the post-retirement years, because of the long latent period for induction of many occupationally-induced cancers.

Occupational cancers are now emerging in countries where the process of industrialization is taking place. For example, high levels of lung cancer have been observed among workers engaged in the manufacture of rubber

41

tyres in some developing countries. Health protection measures in these countries should thus include monitoring the use of potentially carcinogenic materials and processes in industry, providing public education, and enacting appropriate legislation.

Control of occupational cancer

The control of occupational cancer calls for the identification and assessment of existing or potential hazards. Developing countries have an excellent opportunity to learn from the experience of the industrialized countries, and to take steps to avoid the emergence or importation of cancer hazards in

Table 4.2 Selected occupations involving exposure to chemicals, groups of chemicals, industrial processes, or complex mixtures for which there is sufficient evidence to demonstrate carcinogenicity to humans

Industry	Occupation	Site	Causative agent
Agriculture	Vineyard work involving arsenical insecticides	Lung, skin	Arsenic
Extractive (mining)	Uranium mining	Lung	Radon daughters
Asbestos	Mining, manufacture of asbestos-containing products, insulators, etc. Construction work, Ship breaking	Lung, pleural and peritoneal mesothelioma	Asbestos
Petroleum	Shale oil production workers	Skin, scrotum	Polynuclear aromatic hydrocarbons
Metals	Chromium plating	Lung	Chromium
Shipbuilding, motor workers	Shipyard and dockyard workers, motor industry manufacture	Lung, pleural and peritoneal mesothelioma	Asbestos
Chemicals	Vinyl chloride production, dye manufacture and use	Liver angiosarcoma bladder	Vinyl chloride monomer, benzidine, 2-naphthylamine, 4-aminodiphenyl
Gas	Gas workers	Lung, bladder, scrotum	Coal carbonization products, 2-naphthylamine
Rubber	Rubber manufacture	Lymphatic and hematopoietic system (leukaemia)	Benzene
Leather	Boot and shoe manufacture and repair	Nose, bone marrow (leukaemia)	Leather dust, benzene
Furniture	Furniture manufacture and cabinet-making	Nose (adenocarcinoma)	Wood dust
Textiles	Mule spinners	Skin	Mineral oils (containing various additives and impurities)

Source: Tomatis L. et al., eds. *Cancer: causes, occurrences and control.* Lyon, International agency for Research on Cancer, 1990 (IARC, Scientific Publication, No. 100)

industry. Wherever occupational cancer hazards are found to exist, exposure standards must be set that will minimize the risk to workers. This typically requires the appropriate government, scientific, industrial, and labour organizations to review and discuss relevant data and then to agree on controls. Once a quantitative standard is set, industrial processes must be modified to ensure that the agreed maximum exposure level is not exceeded. This may involve the mechanical redesign of a process, substitution of materials, or other significant adaptations. The World Health Organization series *Environmental Health Criteria*, numbering more than 160 monographs, provides guidance on minimizing environmental cancer hazards, including occupational hazards.

Certain industrial processes that demand costly safeguards against exposure to carcinogens are now being exported to countries that are ill equipped to provide those safeguards or to deal with the problems that may arise. International surveillance and control of such situations seem indicated. A valuable source of reference is the list of banned or restricted chemicals and drugs published by the United Nations (New York) and regularly updated: The consolidated list of products whose consumption and/or sale have been banned, withdrawn, severely restricted, or not approved by governments.

Successful control of occupational hazards has been achieved in a number of areas. An excellent example is the modification of manufacturing processes in the dyestuff industry, which substantially reduced the incidence of bladder cancer among workers in the West. Other measures that are valuable in reducing the dangers of unavoidable exposure include the wetting down of potentially carcinogenic particulate matter, to prevent its inhalation; improved ventilation in mines; and use of protective equipment and clothing in many industrial settings.

Cancer control programmes should encourage action at government level to prohibit:

- the importation of hazardous work practices that involve exposure to known carcinogens;
- the dumping of hazardous waste in such a manner that drinking-water or air will become contaminated with carcinogens.

INFECTIONS AND CANCER

Viruses as causative agents

Cancer of the liver is one of the principal human forms of the disease attributable to a virus; chronic infection with hepatitis B or C virus (HBV or

43

HCV) (IARC, 1995). Incidence is particularly high in sub-Saharan Africa and eastern Asia where viral hepatitis (HBV) is transmitted at the time of birth or during early childhood. In Japan, Egypt and for some cases of liver cancer in the United States and Europe, the cause appears to be chronic infection with HCV resulting from past use of unsterilized equipment or contaminated blood products.

The sexually transmitted human papilloma viruses are now recognized as the principal cause of cancer of the uterine cervix, especially subtypes 16 and 18 (IARC, 1995). Infection with these viruses is prevalent in young women, but the factors that cause these infections to persist and in some cases result in the development of invasive cancer are still unknown. Some studies have connected papillomaviruses with cancer of the skin and oral cavity.

A causal relationship has also been observed between Epstein–Barr virus (EBV) and Burkitt lymphoma affecting children in central Africa and in Papua New Guinea, and between EBV and nasopharyngeal carcinoma, especially among populations of southern Chinese origin (IARC, 1997).

AIDS

One of the manifestations of the epidemic of acquired immunodeficiency syndrome (AIDS) is Kaposi sarcoma, a form of cancer that occurs in about 10% of AIDS patients in Europe, North America and Africa, now recognized as being caused by human herpes virus type 8 (IARC, 1997). Another AIDS-related neoplasm is non-Hodgkin lymphoma.

There are three modes of transmission of the human immunodeficiency virus (HIV), the cause of AIDS: sexual; parenteral (through direct inoculation of blood or blood products, for example, in blood transfusions, or by sharing of contaminated needles by intravenous drug users); and perinatal (from an infected woman to her foetus or infant, before, during, or shortly after birth). The principal objective in AIDS control is reduction in HIV transmission through promotion of condom use, provision of sterile needles, access to treatment for drug dependence and prevention of mother-to-child transmission using antiretroviral drugs and/or breastmilk substitutes. The first of these measures is in line with programmes designed to prevent cancer of the uterine cervix, so health educators working in the national cancer control programmes should collaborate with AIDS educators to ensure that messages are compatible and mutually supportive.

Parasitic infections

Schistosomiasis is one of the most widespread human parasitic infections, responsible for a substantial amount of bladder cancer in Egypt, Iraq, and west and south-eastern Africa (IARC, 1994a). The causative organism, *Schistosoma*, passes part of its life cycle in snails that inhabit shallow waters, and is then released into the water, infecting humans by penetrating the skin. Passing of urine or faeces into the water by infected people then continues the life cycle.

A different parasite, the liver fluke, has been shown to give rise to cancer of the bile ducts (cholangiocarcinoma) in south-east Asia and the Korean peninsula (IARC, 1994a).

Bacterial infections

Infection of the stomach lining by a bacterium, *Helicobacter pylori*, known to be a cause of peptic ulcer disease and gastritis, is also a cause of stomach cancer (IARC, 1994a), probably by virtue of its induction of chronic gastritis, recognized to predispose people to stomach cancer. Infection with this bacterium can be eradicated by antibiotic therapy, and it is possible that some of the reduction in stomach cancer in most countries during the 20th century was a result of such therapy. The interaction between infection with *H. pylori* and dietary factors is, however, as yet unresolved, and as indicated above in the discussion of diet, strong associations between diet and stomach cancer are also known and thought to be causal.

Controlling biological agents of cancer causation

Control of cancers induced by biological agents depends upon combating the infection concerned. Essential measures include education to minimize the transmission of infection, for instance teaching people to avoid infected water, unsafe sexual behaviour, injection drug use and sharing of equipment, and urination/defecation in water that will be used by others. Environmental measures, such as eliminating intermediate hosts of the parasites, may be valuable in reducing human exposure. Antiparasitic drugs can successfully treat infestation (and reduce the risk of subsequent cancer), but their use is not a substitute for environmental and personal measures, if the risk of re-infestation remains common.

Effective vaccines would be the most potent weapons against the viruses estimated to cause up to 15% of all cancers. Vaccination is currently available only against the hepatitis B virus. HBV vaccination of infants in areas of high prevalence is being promoted by WHO's Expanded Programme on Immunization as a means of preventing chronic hepatitis. The effect of such vaccination on the incidence of liver cancer should become apparent in about 30 years' time, and there are already some indications that it may be having an effect in reducing liver cancer in young people in Taiwan, China.

Vaccination of injection drug users is another effective measure of preventing the spread of HBV.

Vaccines against the human papilloma viruses that cause cervical cancer are being developed and entering early clinical studies. There is some hope that such vaccines could be effective in those already infected with the virus in preventing the development of cancer (therapeutic vaccines). This could be an additive effect to the usual effect of vaccines against infection, in preventing the establishment of an infection in the first place.

SUNLIGHT

Exposure to excessive ultraviolet radiation from the sun causes all forms of skin cancer (IARC, 1992). Successful education programmes to persuade people to avoid unnecessary exposure to sunlight could dramatically reduce the incidence of both basal cell and squamous cell carcinoma of the skin and probably also of cutaneous melanoma. The main host determinants of susceptibility to melanoma are fair hair and skin. Individuals at high risk are characterized by excessive freckling and benign naevi, with a tendency to burn on exposure to the sun.

The following have been identified as key preventive measures:

- increasing the number of people who are aware of their own risk factors for skin cancer;
- persuading people at high risk to avoid excessive exposure to sun-derived and artificial sources of ultraviolet radiation, and to adopt appropriate protection measures for themselves and their children;
- effecting changes in public attitudes to a tanned appearance.

Promotion of awareness of the hazards of sun exposure by ministries of health and nongovernmental organizations is therefore important in preventing skin cancer. WHO's Intersun Project on ultraviolet (UV) radiation facilitates public and occupational programmes to reduce UV radiation-related health risks, and also develops practical resources in support of those programmes.

The emphasis should be on school programmes aimed at children and young people, because most of lifetime sun exposure occurs during childhood and adolescence. Countries should participate in international agreements to curtail the use of chemicals that damage the earth's ozone layer. In countries where the risk of skin cancer is high, there should be routine monitoring of ultraviolet radiation levels, and the public should be informed whenever levels are particularly high. Avoidance of exposure to the sun between the hours of 11:00 and 15:00 is a sensible precaution.

Use of sunscreens has been controversial. Some studies have suggested that increasing the duration of sun exposure that can be experienced before the skin starts to burn may increase the risk of melanoma and basal cell carcinomas. The use of sunscreens for such purposes should therefore be avoided, and preference should be given to sun avoidance behaviours (IARC, 2000).

SEXUAL AND REPRODUCTIVE FACTORS

The incidence of certain cancers is influenced by a number of sexual and reproductive factors. The risk of breast cancer, for instance, is greater in nulliparous women and in women who have their first child over the age of 25, and especially over age 30. Starting sexual intercourse at a young age and having multiple sex partners have been shown to increase the risk of cervical cancer because of the increased probability of infection with an oncogenic human papillomavirus. Women who have multiple pregnancies incur additional risk, compared to those who have few or none. Women with untreated sexually transmitted infections are also possibly at greater risk of cervical cancer. The use of estrogens to treat menopausal and post-menopausal symptoms produced a significant increase in the incidence of endometrial hyperplasia and cancer, and there is evidence that prolonged use of estrogens by postmenopausal women increases their risk of developing breast cancer (IARC, 1999). This risk seems to disappear after cessation of use for 5 years or more, and is probably outweighed by the beneficial effects on ischaemic heart disease and osteoporosis.

Oral contraceptives are now recognized to increase the risk of breast cancer, at least in young women after prolonged use (IARC, 1999). However, they also reduce the risk of endometrial and ovarian cancer, and the cost–benefit of these combined effects, especially when their other benefits are taken into consideration, justifies their continued use. The use of diethyl-stilbestrol to treat threatened abortion increased the risk of vaginal cancer among the daughters of women so treated (Lanier et al., 1973). It is not known if an increased risk of breast cancer is evident among women who were themselves treated with diethylstilbestrol.

A national cancer control programme should provide education and information on sexual and reproductive factors relating to cancer.

Appropriate topics include:

- the elements of sexual and reproductive behaviour that are risk factors for various forms of cancer (and for sexually transmitted diseases);
- the importance of "safe sex" and the value of barrier methods of contraception;

- family planning to help reduce the risk of cancer of the cervix;
- the risks involved in prolonged use of non-contraceptive estrogens.

Instruction in sexual and reproductive behaviour should start at school. It is important that educational programmes on sexual lifestyles for young people are coherent. Such programmes should emphasize the benefits of protected intercourse in reducing cancer of the cervix, as well as AIDS and other sexually transmitted diseases.

A FRAMEWORK FOR HEALTH PROMOTION

Many factors are involved in cancer control. Therefore, to be more effective, broad based health promotion is required. Health promotion uses an integrated approach, emphasizing partnership, intersectoral collaboration and community participation. The Ottawa Charter for Health Promotion (WHO, 1986c) sets out a strategy with five essential actions (see Box 4.1). Health promotion actions contribute towards:
- developing healthy public policies, legislation, and economic and fiscal controls which enhance health and development, for example on environmental pollution, tobacco control and food safety;
- creating environments that are protective and supportive of health, using mediation and negotiation, for example in relation to asbestos and other carcinogenic substances;

Box 4.1 The Ottawa Charter for Health Promotion

The Ottawa Charter for Health Promotion identifies the following essential actions:

- *building healthy public policy;*
- *creating supportive environments;*
- *strengthening community action;*
- *developing personal skills;*
- *reorienting health services.*

Combinations of the five action areas are the most effective. These actions strengthen capacity and support both individuals and society at large in addressing the social, economic and environmental conditions and specific risk factors that determine health, many of which also impact on cancer control (WHO 1986c).

- strengthening community action through social mobilization, for example gaining acceptance of cancer screening;
- increasing individual knowledge and skills using health education and communication, for example creating awareness of the risk factors in relation to cancer and the importance of cancer screening;
- reorienting health services more towards prevention and consumer needs.

Education, public health policy, and environmental support play key roles in health promotion approaches to cancer control.

Education

As an approach to health promotion, education helps people to make healthy decisions and participate in healthy activities by:
- increasing knowledge and motivation;
- changing attitudes;
- increasing the skills needed to maintain good health.

Health promotion initiatives include a number of educational strategies. One of the most widely used is health communication, the process of promoting health by disseminating information through media channels (for example posters, television, newspapers) or interpersonal contacts.

A number of educational initiatives have the potential to reduce the incidence of cancer and mortality from the disease. Examples include:
- training health professionals to provide counselling on smoking cessation and risks from exposure to environmental tobacco smoke;
- offering classes on healthy food preparation and shopping skills;
- disseminating information on the hazardous effects of excess alcohol consumption, especially in conjunction with tobacco smoking;
- maintaining or initiating efforts to ensure the right of employees to know about hazardous substances in their workplaces;
- adopting public education initiatives to increase awareness of environmental health risks and measures that can be taken to address these risks;
- promoting awareness of the risks of common cancers, and their curability if detected early.

Public health policy

Healthy public policies promote the health of individuals and communities by:
- making it easier to adopt healthy practices;
- making it more difficult to adopt unhealthy practices;

- creating healthy social and physical environments.

There are two main approaches to fostering healthy public policies: health advocacy and community organization. *Heath advocacy* is the process of lobbying decision makers to take action on health-related issues. *Community organization*, often referred to as community development, is the process of mobilizing communities to take action on their shared health concerns. All efforts to facilitate community action should incorporate the process of empowerment, the ability of individuals and communities to control the factors affecting their health.

Some policies that could enhance cancer control include:
- ensuring tobacco is taxed at an appropriate level, and that tobacco taxes are increased at least enough to keep pace with increases in the cost of living;
- introducing legislation banning smoking in the workplace and in schools;
- introducing mandatory warning labels on tobacco and alcohol products;
- enforcing bans on sales of tobacco or alcohol to minors;
- ensuring that alcohol is taxed and alcohol use is banned in the workplace;
- developing a food labelling system that enables consumers to determine the content and nutritional value of food products;
- ensuring that healthy school meals are available to children who need them;
- introducing legislation to reduce the exposure of workers to carcinogens in the workplace;
- ensuring that hepatitis B vaccination is included in expanded programmes of immunization of children in countries with high HBV transmission rates, as well as in immunization programmes for high risk groups such as injection drug users and sex workers.

Environmental support

Environmental support consists of tangible resources, practices and policies that make it easier for people to maintain their health. Some examples of environmental support that helps to reduce the incidence of cancer are:
- smoke-free public places and workplaces;
- ensuring that there is shade in school playgrounds, especially for populations with fair skins;
- encouraging town and residential planning to ensure that people can exercise when they are able;
- provision of adequate levels of income to purchase nutritious food;
- availability of healthy food choices in schools and workplaces;
- workplaces free from hazardous levels of occupational carcinogens;
- pollution-free soil, air and drinking water.

Education, public health policy and environmental support are complementary approaches to health promotion. Each approach can strengthen the impact of the others. All three approaches are necessary to achieve the three purposes of health promotion: health enhancement, risk avoidance and risk reduction.

Health enhancement

Health enhancement reaches the entire population. Health enhancement activities are designed mainly to increase levels of good health, vitality and resilience in all people. Although health enhancement activities may also prevent disease or reduce health risks, their main focus is to enhance health rather than to reduce or prevent illness. For example, a population-based campaign encouraging people to become more physically active is a health enhancement activity that could help to bring about a reduction in the incidence of several forms of cancer, as well as other noncommunicable diseases.

Risk avoidance

Risk avoidance reaches individuals who have not yet developed the health problems associated with a particular health risk. The goal of risk avoidance activities is to ensure that those at low risk of a particular health problem remain at low risk. An effective health education programme aimed at discouraging young people from experimenting with tobacco consumption is one example of how risk avoidance can be applied to prevent cancer and other noncommunicable diseases. A public education campaign pointing out the advantages of locally grown fruits and vegetables and the hazards associated with consumption of high- fat meat products is another.

Risk reduction

Risk reduction reaches those at moderate or high risk of health problems. The goal of risk reduction activities is to modify the environmental conditions, behaviours or predisposing characteristics that are creating the risk for those vulnerable to a particular health problem. Examples of risk reduction activities aimed at preventing cancer include policies to integrate programmes into the primary health care system that will encourage and support smokers who wish to treat their dependence, and to provide early and brief interventions for reducing hazardous or harmful drinking. Other examples include policies to eliminate hazardous emissions of an occupational carcinogen at a work site.

Health promotion activities need to be coordinated, so it may be necessary to appoint a health promotion expert as part of the multidisciplinary team managing the national cancer control programme. This may be particularly necessary when the cancer control activity could be regarded as contrary to the local culture. A particular example is the difficulty many rural women have with the preventive nature of a cervical cancer screening programme, especially those women no longer in contact with maternal and child health services because of their age. Yet, in every community, those older women are at highest risk of cancer of the cervix, and the programme should be especially directed to them.

PRIORITY PREVENTION ACTIONS FOR VARIOUS RESOURCE LEVELS

All countries should give priority to implementing integrated health promotion and prevention strategies for noncommunicable diseases that are consistent with the present and projected epidemiological situation. As a minimum, these interventions should include tobacco prevention and control, reduction of alcohol use, promotion of a healthy diet and physical activity, and education about sexual and reproductive factors.

Furthermore, all countries should establish policies aimed at minimizing occupationally-related cancers, and legislate to control known environmental carcinogenic agents. Strategies should include legislation and regulation, environmental measures, and education at community, school and individual levels.

Avoidance of unnecessary exposure to sunlight should be recommended, particularly in high-risk populations.

Low-resource countries should focus on areas where there are not only great needs, but also the potential for success. They should ensure that priority prevention strategies are targeted to those groups that are influential and can spearhead the whole process, such as policy-makers, health workers, and teachers. In areas with a high prevalence of cancers induced by biological agents, special measures should be developed to combat the infections concerned, for example, schistosomiasis and hepatitis B. In areas endemic for liver cancer, HBV vaccination should be integrated with other vaccination programmes.

Countries with medium levels of resources should consider developing clinical services for brief, effective counselling on tobacco cessation, and other cancer risk factors as well as strengthening education on sexual and reproductive factors. These activities should take place in primary health care settings, schools and workplaces. Medium-resource countries should also consider developing model community programmes for an integrated approach to the prevention of noncommunicable diseases.

Countries with high levels of resources should implement comprehensive, evidence-based health promotion and prevention programmes, and ensure nationwide implementation of these programmes in collaboration with other sectors. Routine monitoring of ultraviolet radiation levels should be established if the risk of skin cancer is high.

EARLY DETECTION OF CANCER

Early detection of cancer is based on the observation that treatment is more effective when the disease is detected earlier in its natural history, prior to the development of symptoms, than in an advanced stage. The aim is to detect the cancer when it is localized to the organ of origin without invasion of surrounding tissues or distant organs.

A decision to implement early detection of cancer in health services should be evidence-based, with consideration for the public health importance of the disease, characteristics of early-detection tests, efficacy and cost-effectiveness of early detection, personnel requirements and the level of development of health services in a given setting. Even if the costs of the screening tests are relatively low, the whole process may involve substantial expenses and may divert resources from other health care activities.

Early detection is only a part of a wider strategy that includes diagnosis, treatment of the condition detected, and follow-up. These activities need to be integrated at appropriate levels of health services, if early detection is to be sustained. Some specific additional investments in health services infrastructure may be required for the extra disease burden resulting from early detection.

There are two principal components of early detection programmes for cancer: education to promote early diagnosis, and screening. Successful education leading to early diagnosis can result in substantial improvement in the health outcome of persons destined to develop cancer. Screening is unlikely to be successful unless based upon an effective education programme and effective treatment for the cancers detected.

Both approaches involve costs to the individual (in terms of time spent, distance travelled, cash payments for detection/diagnosis) and the health services (staff, subsidies for detection/diagnosis, treatment, follow-up), and sometimes may be associated with undesired harm. It is important to establish that benefits of early detection outweigh complications and harmful effects before early detection is implemented as a public health policy. National health services often operate with limited resources against a wide variety of competing priorities. It is essential, therefore, to recommend for implementation only those interventions for which there is sufficient evidence on efficacy and cost-effectiveness.

It is essential to educate people to recognize the early signs and symptoms of cancer. They should understand that cancer, when diagnosed early, is far more likely to be treatable, and to respond to effective treatment. They should appreciate the possible significance of lumps, sores, persistent indigestion or cough, and bleeding from the body's orifices, and the importance of seeking prompt medical attention if any of these occur. The cancers amenable to early diagnosis are: oral cavity, nasopharynx, stomach, colon/rectum, skin melanoma and other skin cancers, breast, cervix, ovary, urinary bladder, and prostate.

Substantial endeavours may be needed in many cultures to dispel the myths, fears and gloom that tend to accompany any consideration of cancer. Otherwise, it is unlikely that the majority of those at risk for cancer will take effective prompt action.

A high proportion of cancers that are relatively curable in developed countries are detected only at advanced stages in developing countries. It is reasonable to assume, therefore, that increased awareness among physicians, allied health care workers, and the general public in developing countries, combined with prompt and effective therapy, could have a major impact on the disease. There is evidence that prompt action, combined with the availability of effective treatment, resulted in improvements in both the stage of cancer at presentation and mortality from cancer of the cervix in developed countries in the last half of the 20th century (Ponten et al., 1995). A similar pattern has become evident more recently in rural India (Jayant et al., 1998).

Professional education of primary health care workers is essential. Such workers are at the forefront of the initial contact between possible cancer patients and the medical care system, and they must be aware of the signs and symptoms of early cancer, even though their prior training may have only exposed them to advanced and often untreatable cancers. This means that they must be systematically trained in the early detection of certain cancers, so that they are alert to the signs and symptoms of early cancer, and they must be given sufficient time to carry out such responsibilities. Further, it may be necessary to improve peoples' accessibility to trained health workers who are competent in performing the necessary examinations (including female health workers for women).

If the majority of common cancers (for example, cervix, breast, mouth, skin) are advanced at presentation (that is, stage III or IV), trained workers should promote measures for earlier diagnosis and referral. Early diagnosis, referral, and treatment of these cancers are of far greater prognostic importance than any attempts to treat the disease in its late stages. Even in cases where the eventual outcome cannot be changed, treatment is simpler and quality of life improved for those cases where early diagnosis is achieved.

Every suspected case of cancer must be promptly referred for appropriate diagnosis and therapy, and institutions with the staff and facilities necessary to provide effective treatment must be accessible to patients. Special measures may be needed to ensure that those referred do in fact attend for diagnosis and management of suspected abnormalities.

SCREENING FOR CANCER

Screening is the presumptive identification of unrecognized disease or defects by means of tests, examinations, or other procedures that can be applied rapidly.

In advocating screening programmes as part of early detection of cancer, it is important for national cancer control programmes to avoid imposing the "high technology" of the developed world on countries that lack the infrastructure and resources to use the technology appropriately or to achieve adequate coverage of the population. The success of screening depends on having sufficient numbers of personnel to perform the screening tests and on the availability of facilities that can undertake subsequent diagnosis, treatment, and follow-up.

A number of factors should be taken into account when the adoption of any screening technique is being considered:
- *sensitivity* – the effectiveness of a test in detecting a cancer in those who have the disease;
- *specificity* – the extent to which a test gives negative results in those that are free of the disease;
- *positive predictive value* – the extent to which subjects have the disease in those that give a positive test result;
- *negative predictive value* – the extent to which subjects are free of the disease in those that give a negative test result;
- *acceptability* – the extent to which those for whom the test is designed agree to be tested.

A screening test aims to be sure that as few as possible with the disease get through undetected (high sensitivity) and as few as possible without the disease are subject to further diagnostic tests (high specificity). Given high sensitivity and specificity, the likelihood that a positive screening test will give a correct result (positive predictive value) strongly depends on the prevalence of the disease within the population. If the prevalence of the disease is very low, even the best screening test will not be an effective public health programme.

It is also important to review the organization of a screening programme (Hakama et al., 1985). The test procedure itself should be efficiently administered. There should also be adequate follow-up of individuals with positive results, so that diagnosis can be quickly confirmed and appropriate therapy started.

Policies on early cancer detection will differ markedly between countries. An industrialized country may conduct screening programmes for cervical and breast cancer. Such programmes are not, however, recommended in the least developed countries in which there is a low prevalence of cancer and a weak health care infrastructure. Further, only organized screening programmes are likely to be fully successful as a means of reaching a high proportion of the at-risk population. Countries that favour cancer detection remaining part of routine medical practice, or that simply encourage people to seek specific tests at regular intervals, are unlikely to realize the full potential of screening.

The success of screening programmes depends on a number of fundamental principles:

- the target disease should be a common form of cancer, with high associated morbidity or mortality;
- effective treatment, capable of reducing morbidity and mortality, should be available;
- test procedures should be acceptable, safe, and relatively inexpensive.

In a national cancer control programme, screening programmes should be organized to ensure that a large proportion of the target group is screened and that those individuals in whom abnormalities are observed receive appropriate diagnosis and therapy. Agreement needs to be reached on guidelines to be applied in the national cancer control programme concerning:

- the frequency of screening and ages at which screening should be performed;
- quality control systems for the screening tests;
- defined mechanisms for referral and treatment of abnormalities;
- an information system that can:
  - send out invitations for initial screening;
  - recall individuals for repeat screening;
  - follow those with identified abnormalities;
  - monitor and evaluate the programme.

For a number of reasons, patients often fail to adhere to recommended cancer screening activities. While in many cases both the patients and the health care providers understand the concept of early detection, they fail to comply with recommendations. Non-compliance is a general health problem and one that should be addressed in a comprehensive manner to improve outcome and reduce the waste of resources.

Screening that concentrates solely on a high-risk group is rarely justified, as identified risk groups usually represent only a small proportion of the cancer burden in a country. In planning the coverage of screening programmes, however, steps must be taken to ensure that all those at high risk are included. This requirement may be difficulty to fulfil. In screening for cancer of the cervix, for example, those at high risk are often difficult to recruit into screening.

The main criteria that should be considered before a screening programme is instituted as part of the national cancer control programme are summarized in Table 5.1.

Screening for cancer of the cervix

Cervical cancer is the second most common cancer among women worldwide, with almost half a million new cases each year (Ferlay et al., 2000). Screening with the cervical smear plus adequate follow-up therapy can achieve major reductions in both incidence and mortality rates (Miller et al., 1990). The smear can reveal cytological abnormalities indicating the presence of a precancerous lesion (various grades of dysplasia, or cervical intraepithelial neoplasia, or low- or high- grade cytological abnormalities, depending on the classification used by the laboratory), as well as *in situ* or very early invasive cancer (see Figure 5.1). Treatment of these early lesions is highly effective, though far more are diagnosed than will ever progress to invasive cancer if untreated.

The experience of the Nordic countries is instructive (Hakama, 1982).

Table 5.1 Criteria for instituting a screening programme

1. The condition to be detected is of public health importance.	**5.** There is sufficient political will, and it is feasible to carry out the relevant screening, diagnostic and intervention practices in a population-based manner with existing resources or with resources that could be obtained during the planning period.
2. The natural history of the condition is understood and there is an unsuspected but detectable (pre-clinical) stage.	
3. There is an ethical, acceptable, safe and effective procedure for detecting the condition at a sufficiently early stage to permit intervention.	**6.** Adoption and implementation of the screening, diagnostic and intervention practices will strengthen development of the health system and overall societal development in a manner consistent with the principles of primary health care.
4. There are ethical, acceptable, safe and effective preventive measures or treatments for the condition when it is detected at an early stage.	**7.** The cost of the screening and intervention is warranted and reasonable compared with alternative uses of resources.

Systematic application of screening in Iceland and Finland during the 1960s sharply reduced cervical cancer in those countries. This contrasts with the slow but steady increase of cervical cancer in Norway, where screening was not applied systematically until 1980, and a lesser decline in incidence in Denmark, where screening programmes were introduced gradually.

Quantitative studies have shown that, after one negative cytological smear for cervical cancer, screening once every three to five years accomplishes about the same effect among women of 35–64 years of age as screening every year (Table 5.2). Even screening once every 10 years yields an important reduction in the incidence of invasive cervical cancer. The bottom half of Table 5.2 shows that the effect in the population will be lower if compliance and sensitivity of the test are less than perfect. Nevertheless, such evidence led a WHO meeting to conclude that countries with limited resources should aim to screen every woman once in her lifetime between 35 and 40 years of age. When more resources are available, the frequency of screening should be increased to every 10 and then every 5 years for women aged 35–55 years (WHO, 1986b). Only when this is achieved, is it legitimate to extend screening to younger ages, and rarely below 25 years of age. Programmatic issues, however, required attention (Miller et al., 2000b).

In the national cancer control programme, wherever laboratories to examine the smears and facilities for treatment of abnormalities are available, the initial aim should be to screen every woman aged 35–40 years once. When 80% of women aged 35–40 years have been screened once, screening frequency should increase to 10-yearly and then 5-yearly for women aged 30–60 years, as resources permit. It is important to recognize that efforts to increase both the quality of laboratory tests, and the compliance of the target population are extremely important, as emphasized by the contrast between the upper and lower parts of Table 5.2. Well organized programmes are, therefore, essential (Hakama et al., 1985). Increasing the frequency of

Fig. 5.1 Screening for cervical cancer

Note: CIN = cervical intraepithelial neoplasia

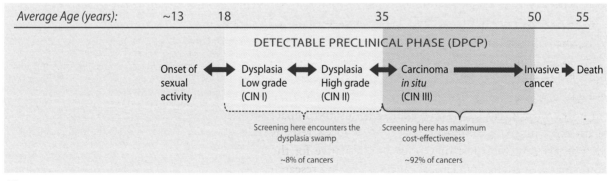

screening or extending screening to younger ages does not compensate for deficiencies in laboratory quality and compliance (Miller, 1992).

In several low resource countries, few laboratory facilities providing good quality cervical cytology are available. This makes it impossible to plan cervical cancer screening using cervical cytology. In such settings, low cost approaches are under investigation. Visual inspection of the cervix with acetic acid application to the cervix (VIA) to help detect precancerous lesions appears to be a promising approach. This is conducted by specially trained health workers using a speculum.

According to the report of a WHO consultation (WHO, 2001a): "The test performance of VIA suggests that it has similar sensitivity to that of cervical cytology in detecting CIN (cervical intraepithelial neoplasia), but has lower specificity. Further research is required to improve its specificity without compromising sensitivity. Information from ongoing studies regarding its longitudinally-derived sensitivity, efficacy in reducing incidence/mortality from cervical cancer, its cost-effectiveness and safety will be useful in formulating public health policies to guide the organization of VIA-based mass population-based screening programmes in developing countries.

It is not known whether cost-savings with a cheap test like VIA might be offset by the referral and investigation of a higher proportion of women who screen positive using this procedure. Since a programme based on VIA involves a certain level of over-treatment, the efficacy, safety and long-term consequences of such a programme also remain to be fully addressed. Thus, information from ongoing studies on these issues will be crucial to judge how appropriate and feasible it will be to introduce VIA-based cervical cancer screening programmes on a population-wide basis in low-income countries." (WHO 2001a)

There is increasing interest in the use of HPV DNA testing for screening, and an international evaluation of the test is under way. Especially for women over the age of 35 years, a negative HPV test could imply that there is no need to screen for 5 or even 10 years. The test, however, requires somewhat sophisticated technical resources, and is not yet ready for routine application within a national cancer control programme. A WHO Consultation (WHO, 2001a) reached the following conclusion: "In middle income countries with some laboratory skills and limited impact of cytology based screening practices, HPV DNA tests as the primary screening test may offer an alternative for the reduction in incidence of cervical cancer. Ongoing research

Table 5.2 Reduction in the cumulative rate of invasive cervical cancer for women aged 35–64 years, with different frequencies of screening

(a) Assuming 100% compliance and a highly sensitive test

Frequency of screening	Percentage reduction in cumulative rate	No. of tests
Yearly	93	30
2-yearly	93	15
3-yearly	91	10
5-yearly	84	6
10-yearly	64	3

Source: Miller AB. (1992) Cervical cancer screening programmes: managerial guidelines. Geneva, World Health Organization.

(b) After correcting for lesser compliance (80%) and reduced sensitivity in practice

Frequency of screening	Percentage reduction in cumulative rate	No. of tests
Yearly	61	30
2-yearly	61	15
3-yearly	60	10
5-yearly	55	6
10-yearly	42	3

should provide data on the cost benefit balance of screening programmes that adopt HPV as a stand-alone screening test. Final proof of the capacity to reduce the incidence of cervical cancer can only be provided by carefully conducted intervention trials."

Screening for breast cancer

Breast cancer is the most common cancer among women worldwide, and there are several possible methods for screening.

If facilities are available, screening by mammography alone, with or without physical examination of the breasts, plus follow-up of individuals with positive or suspicious findings, will reduce mortality from breast cancer by up to one-third among women aged 50–69 years (IARC, In press). Much of the benefit is obtained by screening once every 2–3 years. There is limited evidence for its effectiveness for women 40–49 years of age (IARC, In press)(see Figure 5.2). The Health Insurance Plan (HIP) study, which used physical examinations by surgeons, suggested benefits in younger women only after they had reached their fifties (Shapiro, 1997). A cohort study in Finland suggested breast self-examination to be of benefit at all ages (Gastrin et al., 1994), as did a case-control study in Canada (Harvey et al., 1997). However, observational studies of these latter types cannot exclude selection bias and may overestimate benefit. A randomized trial of breast self-examination in China has not found any evidence of reduction in breast cancer mortality after long-term follow-up (IARC, In press). This suggests that a programme to encourage breast self-examination alone would not reduce mortality from breast cancer. Women should, however, be encouraged to seek medical advice immediately if they detect any change in a breast that suggests breast cancer.

Unfortunately, mammography is an expensive test that requires great

Fig. 5.2 Screening for breast cancer

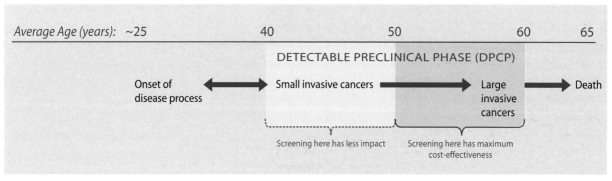

care and expertise both to perform and in the interpretation of results. It is therefore currently not a viable option for many countries. Although there is inadequate evidence that physical examination of the breasts as a single screening modality reduces mortality from breast cancer (IARC, In press), there are indications that good clinical breast examinations by specially trained health workers could have an important role. These come from the HIP study where mammography detected a low proportion of breast cancers, especially in women under the age of 50 (Shapiro, 1997), yet breast cancer mortality was reduced. Similarly, in the Canadian National Breast Screening Study, where the addition of mammography to such examinations in women aged 50–59 did not result in a reduction in breast cancer mortality (Miller et al., 2000a).

Given the present level of evidence, the national cancer control programme should not recommend screening by breast self-examination and physical examinations of the breast. Rather, the programme should encourage early diagnosis of breast cancer, especially for women aged 40-69 years who are attending primary health care centres or hospitals for other reasons, by offering clinical breast examinations to those concerned about their breasts and promoting awareness in the community. If mammography is available, the top priority is to use it for diagnosis, especially for women who have detected an abnormality by self-examination. It should be borne in mind, however, that cancer may be present even if the mammogram is negative. Mammography should not be introduced for screening unless the resources are available to ensure effective and reliable screening of at least 70% of the target age group, that is, women over the age of 50 years.

In determining the relative priorities for different screening programmes, it is important to recognize that breast cancer screening is intrinsically less effective than cytological screening for cervical cancer. As a rough guide, screening will produce an equivalent reduction in numbers of deaths in the two conditions only if, in the absence of screening, breast cancer mortality is three times that of cervical cancer in the age groups concerned.

Screening for colorectal cancer

Evidence to suggest that sigmoidoscopy may be effective for colorectal cancer screening, with benefits lasting for up to ten years, has come from two case-controlled studies (Selby et al., 1992; Newcomb et al., 1992). As such studies cannot eliminate the effect of selection bias, however, this benefit may have been overestimated. Trials are now under way to evaluate flexible sigmoidoscopy and colonoscopy for screening.

Several trials have evaluated the effect of the faecal occult blood test (FOBT). A trial in Minnesota, United States of America, used the FOBT annually in one group and biennially in another. This initially indicated that annual, but not biennial, FOBTs reduce mortality from colorectal cancer after about a ten year period (Mandel et al., 1993). A more recent report, with follow-up for up to 18 years, showed mortality reduction at a lower level from biennial screening (Mandel et al., 1999). Trials in Europe also showed mortality reduction from biennial screening (Hardcastle et al., 1996; Kronborg et al., 1996).

It is clear that a major difficulty with screening using the FOBT is lack of specificity, especially if the test is rehydrated, which substantially increases the costs of programmes. Further, there seems to be a lack in sensitivity for detecting adenomas. Taken together, the FOBT trials suggest that, after an interval of about 10 years, there could be a reduction of up to 20% in colorectal cancer mortality from biennial screening, and a greater reduction as a result of annual screening. Unless high compliance with the test can be achieved, however, the benefit that could be obtained in the general population would be much less, and not commensurate with the expense of the screening programme.

Screening for prostate cancer

Screening for prostate cancer using the digital rectal examination (DRE) is often recommended, but DRE is not a sensitive screening test for early disease. Other screening tests include the prostate specific antigen (PSA) and trans-rectal ultrasound. PSA screening has been widely introduced in the United States, with an initial major increase in the incidence of the disease, and a subsequent reduction. It is not yet clear if such screening reduces the mortality from the disease.

There are many obstacles in the way of an effective screening programme for prostate cancer because of the increasing frequency of latent prostate carcinoma with increasing age and the not inappreciable morbidity and mortality of the radical procedures usually used to treat prostate cancer. It is necessary to establish the effectiveness of screening programmes for prostate cancer by performing well-designed randomized trials, before making any recommendation for public health policy (International Prostate Screening Trial Evaluation Group, 1999). Such trials are underway.

Screening for oral cancer

Early detection (as distinct from organized screening) of oral cancer using visual inspection of the mouth is being considered in countries where incidence is high, such as Bangladesh, India, Pakistan, and Sri Lanka (Sankaranarayanan et al., 2000). The oral cavity is easily accessible for routine examination, and nonmedical personnel can readily detect lesions that are the precursors of carcinoma (WHO, 1984). Furthermore, there are indications that precursor lesions may regress if tobacco use ceases (see Figure 5.3), and that surgical treatment of early oral cancer is very effective. Experience in south-east Asia has demonstrated under field conditions that primary health care workers can examine large numbers of people, and detect and classify precancerous lesions and cancers of the oral region with acceptable accuracy. Some programmes have also encouraged early detection of oral cancer by self-examination using a mirror (Mathew et al., 1995). However, so far it has not been shown that detection of precancerous lesions or early cancers can reduce mortality from the disease.

Screening for cancer at other sites

Where the incidence of stomach cancer is very high, for example, in Japan, a special radiographic technique may be useful in screening (Miller et al., 1990). The technique is expensive, and has so far only been used in Japan.

Screening for lung cancer has been attempted with X-ray and cytological examinations, but investigations have failed to establish its effectiveness (Prorok et al., 1984). Interest has now been raised in the possibility that helical CT scanning may detect lung cancers early (Henschke et al., 1999). The spectrum of cancers detected is, however, unusual (the vast majority are adenocarcinomas), and randomized trials are required before this technique is recommended for adoption.

Because there is an association between melanoma and the presence of numerous skin naevi (moles), systematic self-inspection of the skin could be useful in early detection of this form of skin cancer. Excision and biopsy of naevi that are apparently undergoing malignant transformation might help

Fig. 5.3 Early detection of oral cancer

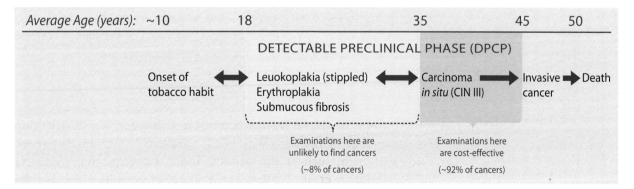

prevent fatalities from the disease, but have not yet been proved effective (Miller et al., 1990).

Where the incidence of bladder cancer is high, for example in areas in which schistosomiasis is endemic or among people who have been occupationally exposed to carcinogens, screening with urinary cytology has been advocated. The value of this technique may be limited, however, because *in situ* lesions may involve a substantial portion of the bladder lining and be difficult to treat (Prorok et al., 1984).

In Chinese populations, with a high incidence of nasopharynx cancer, early cancers can be detected by screening for high levels of certain antibodies to the EBV virus. (IARC, 1997). It is not clear how effective this may be in reducing mortality from the disease.

RECOMMENDED EARLY DETECTION POLICIES FOR VARIOUS RESOURCE LEVELS

Early diagnosis (already symptomatic populations)

As part of a national cancer control programme, all countries should promote awareness of the warning signs for those cancers that display signs and symptoms early in the evolution of the disease. The public should be educated about the changes to watch for, and what to do if they notice these signs. Health workers should be trained to recognize early cancer cases, and refer them rapidly to places where the disease can be diagnosed and treated. Cancer sites amenable to early diagnosis include: oral cavity, larynx, colorectum, skin, breast, cervix, urinary bladder, and prostate (see Table 5.3).

In low-resource settings, low cost and effective community approaches should be used in

Table 5.3 Recommended policies for early detection of selected cancers in health services

Site of cancer	Recommendation for early detection	
	Warning signs	Screening
Oral cavity	Yes	No
Nasopharynx	Yes	No
Oesophagus	No	No
Stomach	Yes	No
Colon/rectum	Yes	No
Liver	No	No
Lung	No	No
Skin melanoma	Yes	No
Other skin cancers	Yes	No
Breast	Yes	Yes
Cervix	Yes	Yes
Ovary	Yes	No
Urinary bladder	Yes	No
Prostate	Yes	No

the first phase to promote early diagnosis of one or two priority detectable tumours. This approach should be adopted initially in a pilot area with relatively good access to diagnosis and treatment.

Countries with medium levels of resources should use low-cost and effective community approaches to promote early diagnosis of all priority detectable tumours.

Countries with high levels of resources should use comprehensive nationwide promotion strategies for early diagnosis of all highly prevalent, detectable tumours.

Screening (asymptomatic populations)

Where level of incidence of the cancer justify it, and the necessary resources can be made available, screening for cancers of the breast and cervix is recommended. This is feasible mainly in medium- and high-resource level countries. Screening for other cancer sites must be regarded as experimental and cannot be recommended at present as public health policy. All countries implementing screening policies should consider the programmatic factors that determine whether or not the programmes achieve effectiveness and efficiency.

In low-resource countries, if there is already infrastructure for cervical cytology screening, the recommendation is to provide high coverage of effective and efficient cytology screening for women 35–40 years old once in their lifetime or, if more resources are available, every 10 years for women 30–60 years old.

Low-income countries that do not have screening facilities should be discouraged from initiating cytology screening. They should wait until the cost-effectiveness of a low cost approach (VIA) is demonstrated.

Countries with medium levels of resources should aim to provide national coverage by cytology screening for cervical cancer at 5-year intervals to women 30–60 years old.

Countries with high levels of resources should reinforce and improve the performance of national screening for cervical cancer and breast cancer if those cancers are common.

DIAGNOSIS AND TREATMENT OF CANCER

6

DIAGNOSIS OF CANCER

The first step in cancer management is to make an accurate diagnosis. This calls for a combination of careful clinical assessment and diagnostic investigations, including endoscopy, histopathology, imaging, cytology, and laboratory studies. Early cancer diagnosis increases the possibility of cure in many, but not all cancers, and reduces the morbidity resulting from the disease and treatment.

Efforts must be made to obtain adequate and appropriate material for cytological or histopathological examination. Relevant clinical information must accompany the material. Light microscopic examination of formalin fixed and haematoxylin and eosin (H & E) stained slides remains the benchmark for histopathological examination. Giemsa's method is the benchmark for haematology. There are few exceptions to the need for histological confirmation before radical management is undertaken.

Cancer diagnosis may be made by direct visualization of the area concerned, for example, by bronchoscopy, oesophagoscopy, mediastinoscopy, colonoscopy, or colposcopy. Even though the tissue appears malignant, a biopsy must be performed to confirm malignancy. Tissue biopsy can be obtained using a fine needle (fine needle aspiration biopsy – FNAB), by a gross needle (core) biopsy, or by total (excisional) or subtotal (incisional) biopsy.

Once a diagnosis is confirmed, it is necessary to undertake further assessment of the patient to ascertain the extent of cancer spread (staging). The goals of cancer staging are:
- to aid in the choice of therapy;
- for prognostication;
- to facilitate the exchange of communication (global communication);
- to determine when to stop therapy;
- to standardize the design of research treatment protocols.

TREATMENT OF CANCER

Treatment should be considered as one component of the national cancer control programme. While the basic principles of treatment are the same throughout the world, the emphasis accorded to treatment will depend upon local patterns of the disease, that is, the commonest types of cancer and the relative proportions of early and late stages. These proportions result not only from prevailing circumstances, but also from the success of early detection and screening programmes for those cancers for which early detection is feasible, affordable and effective. The specific treatment approaches adopted in each country will also depend on the availability of human, physical, and financial resources, as well as the political will to make changes. Decisions on therapies to be offered, and in particular which types of patients should be referred to oncology treatment centres, should preferably be made by a treatment committee designated within the management structure of the national cancer control programme.

The primary goals of cancer treatment are:
– cure;
– prolongation of useful life;
– improvement of quality of life.

Cure in this instance is defined as the attainment of normal life expectancy and has three important components:
– recovery from all evidence of disease (complete remission);
– attainment of a stage of minimal or no risk of recurrence or relapse;
– restoration of functional health (physical, developmental and psychosocial).

In health care, the values that are treasured include autonomy, dignity, prevention of complications of disease, access, justice, cost control, and equity in provision of care. It is important to consider the limitations of cancer therapy in order to avoid expenditure on large treatment centres that serve only a fraction of the population, and deflect resources from areas where they could be used more effectively. Although cure of many common cancers (for example, of the lung and stomach) is not generally possible, curative and palliative treatments are not mutually exclusive. Increasingly, treatment choices will include coordinated curative and palliative elements, evaluated biologically, socioeconomically, and spiritually (see Chapter 7).

Aims and limitations of treatment for cancer

The principal methods of treatment are surgery, radiotherapy, chemotherapy (including hormonal manipulation), and psychosocial support. Although each has a well-established role and can cure some types of cancers, multidisciplinary management is more effective than sequential independent management of the patients. Combined modality approaches result in more cures and improved organ and function preservation. For instance, breast cancers, bone sarcomas and paediatric tumours are now largely treated by combined modalities, and this effects more cures and requires less radical surgery than when single modalities were used. Surgery and radiotherapy are suitable for local and regional disease, and may effect cures in the early stages of cancer, especially when there is an early detection policy. In patients with extensive but localized tumours, surgery and radiotherapy may prove valuable in improving quality of life and potentially in prolonging life. Consideration of their use in such patients must weigh the expected benefits (which will vary with tumour type and stage) against the possible diversion of limited resources from other areas. In general, surgery and radiotherapy have a limited role in the treatment of widely disseminated cancer.

The effectiveness of cancer treatment varies greatly with the site of disease and with a number of social factors. Even within a single country, there may be substantial variation according to such socioeconomic considerations as access to the best available therapy. In some circumstances, it may be appropriate to carry out clinical trials to determine the usefulness of therapy in a particular setting. Such trials should be undertaken only where there are good facilities for data management and where resources are adequate for clinical research.

Except for the surgery of very limited disease or precancer (as for high grade lesions of the uterine cervix), oncological services are dependent on a sound tertiary hospital infrastructure, especially making demands for diagnosis and staging on imaging studies (including, when available, nuclear medicine) and on anatomical pathology and histology.

Role of surgery

Surgery plays an important role in the diagnosis, staging and treatment of local tumours. Even with tumours that show high responsiveness to radiotherapy and chemotherapy, surgery can contribute through removal of tumour masses, palliation and treatment of some complications, such as impending or established pathologic fractures or spinal cord compression. Surgery requires the support of other specialties, including anesthesiology, antibiotic therapy, blood transfusion services, pathology and critical nursing care. The cost-effectiveness of surgery varies according to the stage of disease being treated and, in some patients, the availability of alternative therapies. With early detection programmes, facilities must be available for simple diagnostic and therapeutic surgery at local or district hospitals. Since accurate staging is required in order to limit unnecessary surgery in patients where cure is not possible, reliable diagnostic imaging equipment should be provided. The primary care team must know where and to whom to refer patients with apparently curable malignancies.

The first step for good surgical practice and cancer care is correct diagnosis. Different biopsy techniques (aspiration biopsy, needle biopsy, incisional biopsy, excisional biopsy) should be learned and be performed by well-trained surgeons. Cytopathologic and histopathologic examination requires professional expertise with a strong background in oncopathology.

In many instances, especially with early diagnosis programmes in place, surgery that encompasses a sufficient margin of normal tissue is sufficient therapy. Surgery can effect cures in early stage solid tumours, such as Dukes A or T_1 colon tumours, early prostate, breast, *in situ* (up to stage IIA) carcinoma of the cervix, oral cavity cancers, and early skin tumours, including malignant melanomas, and does not require high technological approaches. Thus surgical skills and facilities for such surgery should be available at the district level. Although some other cancers, such as oesophagus, lung, liver, and stomach, may be cured by surgery alone, the numbers of early stage patients are very small, and their treatment may make large demands on skills and resources.

The objective of surgery for residual disease post chemotherapy or radiotherapy is to provide local cancer control and better chances for adjuvant therapy. The major benefit of such surgery is related to the availability of adjuvant therapy.

Cytoreduction (surgery for debulking) is critical in certain solid tumors, such as ovarian cancer. Except in rare palliative care settings, there is no role for reductive surgery in patients in whom little other effective therapy is possible. Surgery is rarely indicated for metastatic patients (for example, with solitary metastases to lung, liver or brain).

In oncology emergencies, surgery can relieve bowel obstruction, promote cessation of bleeding, close perforations, relieve compression and provide drainage of ascites or pleural effusions. Each category of emergency is unique and treatment must be individualized.

Surgical techniques for reconstruction and rehabilitation can improve function and cosmetic appearance, thus helping to improve quality of life and sometimes restoring patients to occupational activities. Palliative neurosurgical procedures can provide pain relief and relieve functional abnormalities, and thus improve the quality of life of some patients.

Role of radiotherapy

Radiotherapy ranks with surgery as the most important methods of curing local cancer. Radical radiotherapy can effect cures in head and neck cancers, cancer of the cervix, prostate and early Hodgkin disease, and a number of unresectable brain tumours of young people.

Radiotherapy is often administered before surgery (preoperative, neoadjuvant), after debulking surgery with gross residual tumour, or after surgery without clear excision margins (adjuvant) when this surgery is undertaken to preserve function. Radiotherapy either facilitates surgery or consolidates surgical gains, and reduces local recurrence following anal and rectal carcinomas, brain tumours, and breast-conserving surgery for breast cancer.

Palliative radiotherapy is of value in life-threatening situations, such as profuse bleeding from a tumour or the superior vena cava syndrome. Radiation also provides effective palliation in cases of pain secondary to bone metastasis, tumours causing bleeding or compressive syndromes, such as spinal cord compression or cerebral metastatic disease.

Radiotherapy is a capital-intensive specialty, requiring high technology equipment and skilled technicians, found only in tertiary centres. Nevertheless, the costs per patient treated are low if the equipment is used optimally, as most of the costs are initial capital expenditure with relatively low running costs or consumables. Thus savings on personnel, that reduce machine use, increase the costs per patient treated to a level far beyond the savings realized.

If radiotherapy is indicated, the patient may be treated using two broad groups of equipment: teletherapy—treatment from a distance; or brachytherapy—treatment with radioactive sources placed temporarily within body cavities or tissues. For both techniques, quality assurance is essential, with demands on imaging and medical physics services.

Teletherapy may be administered by cobalt machines or by accelerators. Both machines serve the same purpose and the clinical outcomes will be identical. Cobalt machines are less expensive and more robust. The dose rate is predictable and minimal checks are required. Maintenance of machines is simple. The source should be changed at regular intervals of about 5–6 years to keep the treatment time as short as possible. A single dose fraction, or a small number of fractions, will often have an appreciable palliative effect and obliviate the need for protracted therapy schedules.

Accelerators are more expensive and require sophisticated maintenance and frequent calibration. The requirements for stable electrical power and water supplies are high. In the absence of a service contract, breakdowns of major components may incur significant emergency funding. The higher dose rates that accelerators can provide will reduce treatment times, and they will also permit more exact limitation of the fields, but improved imaging, planning and immobilization are required to realize these advantages. A further advantage is the availability of electrons, which are used in about 15% of all radiotherapy patients in advanced radiotherapy departments, especially for the treatment of neck nodes, sparing dose to the spinal cord and skin tumours. For the majority of treatable cancers in developing countries, however, accelerators offer little advantage over cobalt therapy.

To ensure optimal use of teletherapy resources, extended treatment days are advantageous. Two shifts, starting at 06.00 extending to 20.00, are feasible and achievable in some countries.

Brachytherapy may be delivered by a number of different devices: low dose rate (LDR) using caesium and high dose rate (HDR) using iridium or cobalt. LDR is predominantly confined to the treatment of cervical cancer. HDR can be used in the treatment of cervical cancer plus other cancers (for example, nasopharynx and oesophagus), reduces the need for hospital bed occupancy, but demands more expertise and has higher costs.

In planning a national cancer control programme, the accessibility of radiotherapy services in the country has to be carefully considered. A single centre may suffice in small countries, or even in large countries with a small population if transport services between centres of population are adequate. In general, however, a network of oncological services will be required, with a radiotherapy centre within each region of a country. In all eventualities, the treatment committee should define which types of patients should be referred for radiotherapy. For those patients living at a distance from the radiotherapy centre, funding will have to be set aside to pay for the costs of transport and accommodation facilities.

The staffing needs of radiotherapy services should also be reviewed. Where possible, training should be undertaken in programmes with patients, training and equipment relevant to the needs of the country. Radiotherapy staff should be required to obtain a registerable qualification.

Role of chemotherapy

Chemotherapy can effect cures in certain cancers. Even when disease is disseminated, chemotherapy can lead to cures in Hodgkin disease and high grade non-Hodgkin lymphomas, including Burkitt lymphomas, in germ cell tumours, leukaemias and limited stage small cell lung cancer. Chemotherapy is also valuable for palliation in many disease states, including metastatic breast cancer, prostate cancer, and low-grade non-Hodgkin disease. Intensive chemotherapy, such as treatment for lymphomas, requires highly trained physicians. The drugs are expensive and their use demands close monitoring of laboratory tests and skilled nursing support. However, some less toxic chemotherapy agents, such as chlorambucil or prednisolone, and hormonal agents, such as tamoxifen, can be given in primary or district level treatment centres.

Adjuvant therapy is treatment given in addition to primary definitive therapy in the absence of macroscopic residual disease. The goal is to avoid metastases, prolong life, and improve quality of life. Adjuvant chemotherapy and endocrine therapy have been shown to prolong life in breast cancer, while adjuvant chemotherapy has been shown to be of value in colorectal cancers.

Neoadjuvant (induction) chemotherapy has proved useful in osteogenic sarcomas. Clinical trials are under way to ascertain its usefulness in head and neck tumours and in breast cancer.

Tumours can be categorized in terms of their curability (Table 6.1):

- Category 1 tumours are those for which there is evidence that the use of one drug, or a combination of drugs, alone or in conjunction with other therapeutic measures, will result in the cure of at least some patients.
- Category 2 tumours are those where the average survival is prolonged when chemotherapy is used as an adjuvant to surgery or radiotherapy in the early stages of disease.
- Category 3 tumours are those for which there is evidence that the use of a single drug or combination of drugs will cause tumour shrinkage and possibly improvement in the quality of life; survival may be prolonged, but this may be of short duration.
- Category 4 tumours are those where local control may be improved by the use of chemotherapy before, during or after surgery or radiotherapy.
- Category 5 tumours are those for which there are currently no effective drugs. Although some drugs have been shown to cause a degree of tumour shrinkage, the effect is so marginal that quality of life is unlikely to be improved in any but extremely rare instances, and is more likely to be compromised; survival time of patients with category 5 tumours may even be shortened by chemotherapy.

More than 100 cytotoxic drugs are currently available. WHO has established a list comprising 17 drugs that, on the basis of their cost-effectiveness and life-saving potential, are needed to treat the 10 most common cancers or category 1 or 2 cancers (Sikora et al., 1999) (Table 6.2). This list of drugs should form the basis of national policies concerning the chemotherapy to be offered in the light of the

Table 6.1 Categorization of tumours in terms of their curability with chemotherapy or hormone therapy

Category 1 – Curative

Germ-cell cancers	Trophoblastic cancers
Acute lymphoblastic leukaemia	Acute myeloid leukaemia
Acute promyelocytic leukaemia	Hairy-cell leukaemia
Hodgkin disease	Non-Hodgkin lymphoma

Category 2 – Adjuvant

Breast cancer	Colorectal cancer (Dukes C)
Ovarian cancer	Osteosarcoma
Ewing sarcoma	Neuroblastoma
Retinoblastoma	Soft tissue sarcoma
Wilm tumour	

Category 3 – Palliative

Small-cell lung cancer	Non-small-cell lung cancer
Chronic lymphocytic leukaemia	Chronic myelogenous leukaemia
Anal cancer	Bladder cancer
Endometrial cancer	Prostate cancer
Kaposi sarcoma, non-HIV	Oesophageal cancer
Indolent AIDS-related	Head and neck cancer
lymphoma and Kaposi sarcoma	Stomach cancer
Cervical cancer	

Category 4 – Neoadjuvant

Oropharyngeal cancer	Nasopharyngeal cancer

Category 5 – Ineffective

AIDS-related central nervous	Hepatobiliary cancers
system lymphoma	Pancreatic cancer
Melanoma	Thyroid cancer
Renal cell cancer	Central nervous system cancers

Source: Sikora K. et al. Essential drugs for cancer therapy. *Annals of Oncology*, 1999, 10:385–390

cancer problem in the country concerned. Generic forms of these drugs are available, though confirmation of their biological activity is essential.

Development of a treatment policy

It is important to underscore the close link between early detection and treatment. An excellent screening programme would be inappropriate without effective treatment measures. Similarly, it is not useful to develop treatment capacity without encouraging early detection.

The application of effective treatment policies requires a "team" approach in which social workers and family members, as well as health care professionals, provide specific and supportive care for patients with cancer. Education of the patient and family members should thus be considered as components of the management of cancer.

The development of a treatment policy as part of the national cancer control programme requires the establishment of a treatment subcommittee, chaired by a member of the cancer control programme committee. All relevant health care professions should be represented on the subcommittee; membership should therefore include a radiotherapist, surgeon, chemotherapist, nurse, and social worker. Since treatment policy will depend on the predominant forms and stages of cancer and the available resources, epidemiologists and representatives of the health ministry should either become permanent members of the subcommittee or provide relevant information to the subcommittee, such as information on the predominant types and stages of cancer in the geographical region concerned.

The treatment subcommittee should set specific targets, so that progress in the establishment and implementation of the national cancer control programme can be measured. These may include short-term goals,

Table 6.2
Essential drugs for oncology and their indications

Drug	Top 10 cancers	Category 1 or 2 tumours
Bleomycin	+	+
Chlorambucil	+	+
Cisplatin	+	+
Cyclophosphamide	+	+
Doxorubicin	+	+
Etoposide	+	+
5-Fluorouracil	+	+
Methotrexate	+	+
Prednisolone	+	+
Procarbazine		+
Tamoxifen	+	+
Vinblastine	+	+
Vincristine	+	+
Cytarabine		+
Dactinomycin		+
Daunorubicin		+
6-Mercaptopurine		+

Source: Sikora K. et al. Essential drugs for cancer therapy.
Annals of Oncology, 1999, 10: 385–390

such as the establishment of treatment guidelines for specific cancers, and longer-term goals, such as the collection of data that allow measurement of the success of the treatment policy. Guidelines for treatment of each stage of each cancer should be established, based on realistic estimates of the chance of cure, as well as the availability of resources. For example, in early cervical cancer, since there is no evidence to show whether surgery or radiotherapy produces the better outcome, the recommended treatment may depend upon the availability and expected use of surgical and radiotherapy resources for other major tumours in the region. Even when a particular method of treatment has been shown to be superior, a less effective method might still be legitimately chosen if it leads to more efficient overall use of resources and ultimately to greater success in saving lives or improving the quality of life. At all times, allocation of resources should give precedence to patients with the highest potential for cure over those with incurable or probably incurable tumours, who should be identified for palliative care (Table 6.3).

Table 6.3 Five-year relative survival (%) for all stages of cancer of various sites in cases diagnosed in the United States of America (whites), Europe, and the range for developing countries

It is more cost-effective to treat with curative intent cervix, breast, oral cavity, and colon cancers than lung, liver, stomach, and oesophagus, as in the latter group all modalities are largely ineffective, especially for advanced disease (Table 6.4). Stage by stage, treatment is as effective in the elderly as the young, though clearly the potential years of life gained are greater for the young than the old, and as the old have more co-morbidity, treatment will be tolerated better by the young. With the information currently available, the following cost-effective policy guidelines can be suggested:

- Use existing referral systems to provide treatment for patients with early stage tumours that are potentially curable, as for example of the cervix, breast, oral cavity, and colorectal cancers.

Site of cancer	USA (white)		Europe 1985–1989[1]		Developing countries[2]
	1974–1986	1986–1991	Males	Females	1982–1992
Oesophagus	9.4	12.7	7.4	12.2	3.3–26.5
Stomach	16.8	19.5	19.3	23.6	7.5–28.2
Colon	55.2	62.5	46.8	46.7	29.1–45.4
Rectum	53.9	61.8	42.6	42.9	22.6–45.7
Liver	6.5	10.3	4.6	4.7	0.6–12.9
Pancreas	4.2	5.6	4.1	3.9	2.5–7.2
Lung	14.6	15.7	8.9	9.9	3.2–13.8
Skin melanoma	81.5	87.2	68.2	81.4	39.2–47.0
Breast (Females)	76.1	83.6		72.5	44.1–72.7
Cervix	68.2	70.1		61.8	28.0–64.9
Corpus uteri	88.8	88.2		73.2	58.7–76.7
Ovary	45.1	53.2		32.9	33.6–45.0
Prostate	75.3	88.9	55.7		34.5–45.9
Bladder	81.1	86.1	65.2	59.7	23.5–66.1
Kidney	56.4	64.0	47.7	49.3	19.1–49.2
Hodgkin disease	77.3	79.6	70.7	73.1	30.5–59.0
Non-Hodgkin lymphoma	55.7	54.2	45.2	48.4	17.7–37.4
Leukaemia	39.9	48.1	33.5	35.3	4.7–22.6

1 *Source:* Berrino F. et al., eds. *Survival of cancer patients in Europe: the EUROCARE-2 Study.* Lyon, International Agency for Research on Cancer, 1999 (IARC Scientific Publications, No. 151).

2 *Source:* Sankaranarayanan R., Black R.J., Parkin D.M., eds. *Cancer survival in developing countries.* Lyon, International Agency for Research on Cancer, 1998 (IARC Scientific Publications, No. 145)

- Refer children and young adults with leukaemia, lymphoma, brain and germ cell tumours to tertiary centres where they can optimize their chances of cure.
- Provide cheap oral drugs, such as tamoxifen, for metastatic breast cancer at primary levels.
- Provide supportive care facilities and centres for pain management for the majority of cancers that are incurable. These facilities should be community-based, and staffed by community members. Most of the activities should be undertaken on an out-patient basis. If possible, facilities for the terminally ill should be made available.

Development of a follow-up policy

Some cancers may need regular reviews at a referral or a specialist cancer centre, while others can be adequately reviewed and followed up by the family physician or general practitioner or even a physician assistant or clinical assistant. These health care professionals need to be made aware of what to look for at each follow-up visit and what should prompt referral to a specialist at a referral or a cancer centre. Follow-ups can be labour-intensive, and they may provoke unnecessary anxiety. The follow-up policy and guidelines should depend on the types of cancers commonly seen in a given region or country and the resources available (human, material, and fiscal), as well as on the medico-legal requirements regarding irradiated patients. Such guidelines should specify the tests to be performed at each visit.

Table 6.4 Various approaches to treatment of common cancers, taking into consideration biology, stage on presentation, combined therapies, applicability in developing countries, and other prognostic factors

CANCER	Early detection	Surgery	Radiation	Chemotherapy/ hormonal adjuvant therapy	Neoadjuvant therapy	Palliative care
Mouth/ Pharynx	+	++	+++	+	–	+++
Oesophagus	–	+	++	–	–	+++
Stomach	+	+	–	–	–	+++
Colon/ Rectum	++	+++	++	+++	–	+++
Liver	–	+	–	–	–	+++
Lung	–	+	++	–	–	+++
Breast	+++	+++	++	+++	–	+++
Cervix	+++	++	+++	–	–	+++

Key: – = no role; + = small role; ++ = modest role; +++ = major role

Development of referral policies

Efficient implementation of the treatment policy will require careful consideration of the health system organization and distribution of resources, and the establishment of clear guidelines on referral between the various levels of treatment centres in the region. Triage of patients is essential at the time of initial referral: decisions must be made on whether to undertake comprehensive evaluation with a view to therapy (if this is feasible) or to provide palliative care. For each form of cancer, tumours that are considered to be curable in a high proportion of cases, those curable in a lower proportion of cases, and those that are incurable must be clearly identified, and optimal specific treatment or palliative care defined for each. Where resources are inadequate to treat the expected numbers of patients in these categories, the treatment subcommittee may either request additional resources or modify the treatment approach, for example by reducing the number of radiotherapy treatments, accepting a minor reduction in efficacy in order to treat more patients within a given period of time. In general, the more limited are the available resources, the greater should be the emphasis on outpatient treatment, short-duration therapy, and radiotherapy or surgery without chemotherapy. With respect to policy on chemotherapy, it may be advantageous to use the same treatment protocol for several diseases, for example, 5-fluorouracil or a combination of drugs such as 5-fluorouracil and etoposide for all cancers of the upper gastrointestinal tract in which adjuvant therapy is deemed appropriate.

Decisions on the potential for curative therapy need to be made at the primary care level. It is pointless to refer a patient to a major hospital centre if all that can be offered there is palliative care. However, once a decision has been made to refer a potentially curable patient, there should be some means of ensuring that he or she does in fact attend the treatment centre, otherwise the potential for cure will be lost. This is particularly critical for patients identified as a result of early diagnosis or screening programmes.

Within the national cancer control programme guidelines should be established for integrating treatment resources with early diagnosis and screening programmes, and for providing optimal therapeutic management of the most frequently occurring cancers. The management guidelines should specify essential treatments according to the curability of the disease, coverage of patients by available types of therapy, and analysis of the cost-effectiveness of the various approaches.

Compliance

The effectiveness of treatment can be drastically reduced due to poor compliance with therapy. Poor compliance negatively affects health outcomes while increasing health care costs. Factors that influence the rate of compliance include the patient, the health-care team, illness and treatment, and the health system. WHO is currently developing a cost-effective, comprehensive set of strategies to improve compliance (adherence), for inclusion as a routine component of health care for all patients.

Psychosocial services

For those diagnosed with cancer, psychosocial services should be available and should include the assessment of patients for the presence of anxiety and depression, support to help patients adhere to treatment plans, skill building for coping with cancer stress and basic emotional support. For those with clinical range anxiety or depression, care should be available to help ameliorate symptoms. Psychosocial support should also be available for families of cancer patients and staff members who treat cancer patients.

Rehabilitation

Physical, psychological and social rehabilitation aims at improving the quality of life of persons with impairments due to cancer by assisting them to recover their ability to perform everyday activities to live as independently as possible. The type and intensity of the rehabilitation depends on the type and severity of the impairment, and the type and magnitude of the treatment provided. The characteristics of the person and the social environment are also important factors determining the nature of rehabilitation. In general terms, physical and psychological rehabilitation should be provided as early as possible after treatment and within the community where the person lives. Rehabilitation should include support for mobility, self-care, emotional well being, spirituality, vocational pursuits and social interactions.

Some ethical considerations in cancer treatment

Important ethical principles to consider when treating cancer are autonomy and distributive justice. Respect for patients' autonomy necessitates that they be given the opportunity to make choices. However, the disclosure of information to allow for truly informed consent, as is demanded by most developed countries, is not universally accepted and caregivers need to be sensitive to, and respect the values of their patients, especially if they are from different cultural backgrounds. Equitable distribution of resources is an important ethical concern in cancer treatment. The equipment and drugs are both expensive and likely to consume a large component of the health care budget, sometimes for only a few patients (e.g. bone marrow transplantation). The role of the care professional is no longer only to act as an advocate for the individual patient, but as much a gatekeeper of resources for the entire population. For instance, local preferences might be for the use of scarce resources to treat a form of cancer that is relatively uncommon, but for which there is a good chance for cure, as is the case with Burkitt lymphoma in some parts of Africa. Alternatively, local values may dictate that resources be directed in the management of tumours that are common, though incurable, and therefore the provision of palliative care facilities would be given precedence. These considerations should also take account of the problems that may arise with the use of treatments that rely on advanced technology. If such technology is imported from developed countries into less developed areas, due regard should be taken of local circumstances, and for the need for medical and technical personnel trained in its use.

PRIORITY ACTIONS FOR CANCER TREATMENT ACCORDING TO RESOURCE LEVELS

All countries should ensure the accessibility and effectiveness of diagnosis and treatment services by establishing evidence-based clinical and management guidelines, an essential drugs list, good referral, follow-up and evaluation systems, and continuous training of the different health professionals involved. Furthermore, guidelines should emphasize the avoidance of offering curative therapy when cancer is incurable, and patients should be offered palliative care instead.

Countries with low or medium levels of resources should organize diagnosis and treatment services to give priority to common, early detectable tumours, or to those with high potential for cure.

Countries with a high level of resources should reinforce the development of comprehensive cancer treatment and palliative care centres that are especially active for clinical training and research, and that can act as reference centres within the country as well as at the international level.

Pain Relief and Palliative Care

7

As in other fields of medicine, palliative care for cancer patients has progressed over the past decade. The earlier WHO definition of palliative care stressed its relevance to patients not responsive to curative therapy (WHO, 1990b). This statement might be interpreted as relegating palliative care to the last stages of care. Today, however, there is wide recognition that the principles of palliative care should be applied as early as possible in the course of any chronic, ultimately fatal illness. This change in thinking emerged from a new understanding that problems at the end of life have their origins at an earlier time in the trajectory of disease. Symptoms not treated at onset become very difficult to manage in the last days of life. People do not "get used to" cancer pain; rather, chronic unrelieved pain changes the status of the neural transmission of the pain message within the nervous system, with reinforcement of pain transmission, and activation of previously silent pathways.

Symptoms not only influence quality of life, but also influence the course of disease. Pain can kill (Liebeskind, 1991), and so can depression (Wulsin, 2000). Cachexia either directly accounts for the deaths of millions of patients each year, or serves as a major contributory cause (Tisdale, 1997). These symptoms are associated with a chronic stress reaction characterized by aberrations in cytokine production (Dunlop, Campbell, 2000) and activation of the neuroendocrine-hypothalamic systems. Unregulated cytokine production adversely affects many symptoms common in cancer patients, and can enhance tumour progression (Dunlop, Campbell, 2000). Therefore, impeccable control of symptoms throughout the course of illness may have an impact not only on quality of life, but also on length of life, through mediation of the cytokine–stress reaction associated with symptoms.

WHO DEFINITION OF PALLIATIVE CARE

Palliative care is an approach that improves the quality of life of patients and their families facing the problem associated with life-threatening illness, through the prevention and relief of suffering by means of early identification and impeccable assessment and treatment of pain and other problems, physical, psychosocial and spiritual. Palliative care:

- provides relief from pain and other distressing symptoms;
- affirms life and regards dying as a normal process;
- intends neither to hasten or postpone death;
- integrates the psychological and spiritual aspects of patient care;
- offers a support system to help patients live as actively as possible until death;
- offers a support system to help the family cope during the patient's illness and in their own bereavement;
- uses a team approach to address the needs of patients and their families, including bereavement counselling, if indicated;
- will enhance quality of life, and may also positively influence the course of illness;
- is applicable early in the course of illness, in conjunction with other therapies that are intended to prolong life, such as chemotherapy or radiation therapy, and includes those investigations needed to better understand and manage distressing clinical complications.

A continuum of care associated with palliative care is described graphically in Figure 7.1. Therapy intended to modify the disease declines as the illness progresses. The provision of palliative care increases as the person nears the end of life and provides support for the family during this entire period. After the patient dies, bereavement counselling for family and friends is also important.

The quality of life dimensions of palliative care are illustrated in Figure 7.2. Palliative care is concerned with not only all aspects of the patient's needs, but also the needs of the family and of the health care providers.

Figure 7.1
Continuum of Care

Adapted from:
American Medical Association.
Institute for Medical Ethics (1999)
EPEC: education for physicians on end-of-life care. Chicago, Ill: American Medical Association: EPEC Project, The Robert Wood Johnson Foundation.

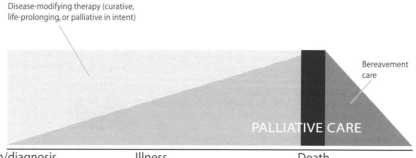

Disease-modifying therapy (curative, life-prolonging, or palliative in intent)

Bereavement care

PALLIATIVE CARE

Presentation/diagnosis   Illness   Death

WHO DEFINITION OF PALLIATIVE CARE FOR CHILDREN

Palliative care for children represents a special, albeit closely related field to adult palliative care. WHO's definition of palliative care appropriate for children and their families is as follows; the principles also apply to other paediatric chronic disorders (WHO, 1998a):

- Palliative care for children is the active total care of the child's body, mind and spirit, and also involves giving support to the family.
- It begins when illness is diagnosed, and continues regardless of whether or not a child receives treatment directed at the disease.
- Health providers must evaluate and alleviate a child's physical, psychological, and social distress.
- Effective palliative care requires a broad multidisciplinary approach that includes the family and makes use of available community resources; it can be successfully implemented even if resources are limited.
- It can be provided in tertiary care facilities, in community health centres and even in children's homes.

Medicine has always emphasized early recognition of a problem in order to alleviate it or prevent its full development. Similarly, palliative care should be recognized as an exercise in prevention—prevention of ultimate suffering through prioritizing the diagnosis and skilful management of sources of distress, both in the form of physical symptoms and of psychosocial and spiritual concerns, at the earliest possible moment (MacDonald, 1991).

The acceptance of the integral role of palliative care in the management of cancer, AIDS and other noncommunicable and ultimately fatal disorders, will enhance its overall understanding and support by the community, political leaders, and health professionals alike.

Figure 7.2 Quality of life dimensions of palliative care

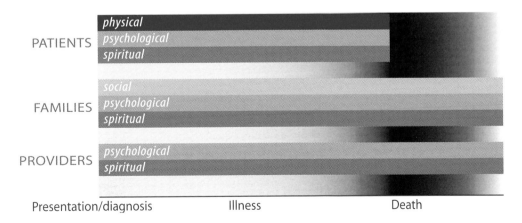

PATIENTS
- physical
- psychological
- spiritual

FAMILIES
- social
- psychological
- spiritual

PROVIDERS
- psychological
- spiritual

Presentation/diagnosis   Illness   Death

RELEVANCE

Despite an overall 5-year survival rate of nearly 50% in developed countries, the majority of cancer patients will need palliative care sooner or later. In developing countries, the proportion requiring palliative care is at least 80%. Worldwide, most cancers are diagnosed when already advanced and incurable (WHO, 1990b).

As discussed in Chapter 3, the incidence and mortality of cancer and of other noncommunicable diseases will increase in the next 20 years. For millions of people, access to palliative care will be the core essential need.

Patients with AIDS, and chronic, ultimately fatal, noncommunicable disorders other than cancer suffer with problems similar to those commonly encountered in cancer patients. Pain, dyspnoea, wasting, confusional states, psychosocial distress, and other devastating symptoms commonly afflict AIDS patients and those with chronic noncommunicable diseases. As symptom etiology (AIDS wasting is a possible exception) is often common across diseases, the principles of palliative care apply across a broad spectrum of disorders. As the roots of suffering in different disorders are common, palliative care programmes must prepare to enrol patients with a wide range of chronic, potentially fatal disorders. This principle is already well represented in paediatric palliative care. This tenet also underlines the importance of cooperation between programmes on cancer, AIDS and noncommunicable diseases to cooperate in the joint development and support of palliative care initiatives.

RESOURCE ALLOCATION

The fundamental responsibility of the health profession to ease the suffering of patients cannot be fulfilled unless palliative care has priority status within public health and disease control programmes; it is not an optional extra. In countries with limited resources, it is not logical to provide extremely expensive therapies that may benefit only a few patients, while the majority of patients presenting with advanced disease and urgently in need of symptom control must suffer without relief.

Throughout the world, governments, medical-nursing societies and nongovernmental organizations have expressed strong support for WHO's definitions of palliative care, and have endorsed the integration of their principles into public health and disease control programmes. Despite this acceptance, a yawning gap is evident between rhetoric and realization. A national disease control plan for AIDS, cancer and noncommunicable disorders cannot claim to exist unless it has an identifiable palliative care component.

ASSESSMENT

Patients with advanced cancer suffer from multiple symptoms that need to be assessed and charted on a regular basis. This is essential for individual patient care, and as an outcome measure for programme development and evaluation. Simple numeric, verbal, or visual analogue measurement of symptoms has been recognized as an essential component of good palliative care.

Care of the dying extends beyond pain and symptom relief. It also supports the social, psychological and spiritual needs of the patients and their families. Therefore it is important to assess these needs and be able to respond with a holistic approach.

DRUG AVAILABILITY

A palliative care programme cannot exist unless it is based on a rational national drug policy. This policy must include the following elements:
- acceptance of the WHO essential drug list (Sikora, 1999);
- regulations that allow ready access of suffering patients to opioids—this may require licensing of specially trained nurses;
- fair pricing by the pharmaceutical industry—this should include access to essential drugs produced at low cost in developing countries, and inter-country or regional buying arrangements;
- a logistic plan for equitable in-country distribution;
- emphasis on training within professional schools on the application of the essential drugs.

EDUCATION

Education in pain relief and palliative care must be an essential component of training for all health workers who may be expected to treat patients with advanced chronic illness. In this regard, there is a need for guidance by ministries of health, backed up by regulations if necessary. Implementation of pain relief and palliative care measures would have a major impact on the quality of life of patients, but will not happen without strong political motivation and leadership (Stjernswärd, 1993). An example of a training programme is the Education for Physicians on End-of-life Care (EPEC) Project developed by the American Medical Association in the United States (American Medical Association. Institute for Ethics, 1999).

GOVERNMENT POLICY

The government of each WHO Member State has a responsibility to establish a national policy and programme for pain relief and palliative care. Policy elements include measures to:

- ensure that the palliative care programme is incorporated into the existing health care system;
- ensure that health workers are adequately trained in cancer pain relief and palliative care;
- ensure that equitable support is provided for programmes of palliative care, particularly in the home, and revise national health policies if necessary;
- ensure that hospitals are able to offer appropriate specialist back-up and support for home care;
- ensure the availability of opioid, nonopioid, and adjuvant analgesics, particularly morphine, for oral administration.

COMPONENTS OF PALLIATIVE CARE

Pain relief

Relief from cancer pain can be achieved in about 90% of patients (United States Department of Health and Human Services, 1994). The main obstacles to pain relief in cancer are insufficient availability of opioid drugs, because of regulatory and pricing obstacles, ignorance, and false beliefs. In order to overcome these interrelated problems, a pain relief programme should be established within the broader palliative care programme. Policymakers therefore need to:

- identify and acknowledge the problem;
- be aware that the problem can be addressed using inexpensive drugs;
- define policy aims and goals;
- ensure that specific resources are available for cancer pain relief;
- examine resources available at the primary care level, and ensure that doctors and nurses are aware of the resources available and know how to obtain access to them.

Freedom from cancer pain must be regarded as a human rights issue (WHO,

1998b). Unrelieved pain in cancer patients is unacceptable because it is generally avoidable (see Box 7.1). The WHO cancer pain relief programme calls for:

- the establishment of a global network to disseminate knowledge of what can be done;
- increased public awareness that pain is almost always controllable;
- incorporation of cancer pain management in the undergraduate and post-graduate training of doctors and nurses;
- inclusion of pain management in standard cancer textbooks;
- treatment of cancer pain in general hospitals, in health centres and at home—not only in oncology departments and cancer centres;
- revision of national drug legislation to facilitate the availability of analgesic drugs to patients;
- additional funds from public and private sources to support local and national cancer pain relief programmes.

WHO has produced several publications on policies and guidelines for cancer pain relief and other aspects of palliative care (WHO, 1990b, 1996, 1998a, 1998b). National cancer control programmes should include responsibility for:

- distribution of the WHO guidelines to all relevant health workers and administrators;
- translation of the WHO guidelines into a form that is suitable for family members and non-medical personnel involved in palliative care;

Box 7.1 WHO Ladder for Cancer Pain

WHO has developed a relatively inexpensive yet effective method for relieving cancer pain in about 90% of patients. This method is called the WHO ladder for cancer pain relief, and it can be summarized in five phrases:

"By mouth"
Whenever possible analgesics should be given by mouth in order to permit wide applicability of this method.

"By the clock"
Analgesics should be given by the clock, that is, at fixed intervals of time. The next dose should be given before the effect of the previous one has fully worn off, to relieve pain continuously.

"By the ladder"
The first step in the ladder is a non-opioid, typified by aspirin. If this does not relieve the pain, an opioid for mild to moderate pain, typified by codeine, should be added as the second step of the ladder. If this fails to relieve the pain, an opioid for moderate to severe pain, typified by morphine, should be used as the third step of the ladder. Additional drugs, called adjuvants, are used under certain conditions. For example, psychotropic drugs are used to calm fears and anxiety.

"For the individual"
There is no standard dose for opioid drugs. The "right" dose is the dose that relieves the patient's pain.

"Attention to detail"
The need for regular administration of pain-relief drugs should be emphasized. Ideally, the patient's drug regimen should be written out in full for the patient and family to work from.

- provision for training doctors and other health workers in the elements of palliative care and the WHO three-step analgesic ladder (see Figure 7.3);
- ensuring that drug regulators give full consideration to the availability of analgesics, notably oral morphine, and amend regulations which inhibit their use for cancer pain management;
- ready availability of analgesics at a cost that ensures that no patient, however poor, will be deprived of access to necessary drugs;
- home care for patients with advanced cancer;
- hospitals in offering appropriate back-up and support.

Psychological support

Good communication is the key to psychological support. Imparting information must be undertaken with honesty and openness, in an atmosphere of sensitivity and compassion, with adequate emotional support (Buckman, 1996). The level of information and pace at which it is given should be appropriate for an individual's ability, needs and culture.

Usually, patients want information on their illness (Centano-Cortes, Nunez-Olarte, 1994; Faulkner, Peace, O'Keeffee, 1993; Meredith et al., 1996; Sell et al., 1993; Simpson et al., 1991), but, in many parts of the world, information with ominous portent is withheld from patients. While this practice is based on compassion and family concern, a 'conspiracy of silence' and a 'conspiracy of words' may add to a patient's suffering. Progressive acceptance by the patient of what is happening often occurs naturally and slowly, in a truly supportive environment. Unless patients are enabled to unburden themselves and share their anxieties and fears, pain and other symptoms may become the intractable avenue through which psychosocial distress is expressed (Twycross, 1994).

Although it may be impossible to offer hope of a cure, it is always possible to offer pain relief, psychosocial support, improved

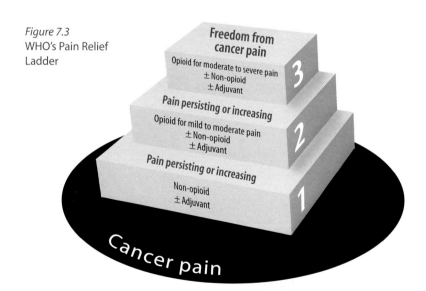

Figure 7.3
WHO's Pain Relief Ladder

quality of life, and comfort in dying. However, as with pain management, there is a need for specific training in communication skills (Faulkner et al., 1995).

Involving the family

The word "family" is used in a broad sense to include actual relatives and other people important to the patient. The role of families in palliative care is very important. Patients and families may have little knowledge of the disease and its prognosis, and may have low expectations of pain relief or unrealistically high expectations of anticancer treatment. Every effort should be made to empower the patient and family by:

- involving them in decision-making with regard to treatment;
- explaining treatments in such a way that they can give informed consent (or informed refusal);
- facilitating a continuing sense of their being in control by providing appropriate advice and practical support.

PRIORITY ACTIONS FOR PALLIATIVE CARE ACCORDING TO RESOURCE LEVELS

All countries should implement comprehensive palliative care programmes with the purpose of improving the quality of life of the majority of patients with cancer, or other life-threatening conditions, and their families. These programmes should provide pain relief, other symptom control, and psycho-social and spiritual support. All countries should promote awareness among the public and health professionals that cancer pain can be avoided, and should ensure the availability of oral morphine in all healthcare settings.

In low-resource settings it is important to ensure that minimum standards for pain relief and palliative care are progressively adopted at all levels of care in targeted areas, and that there is high coverage of patients through services provided mainly by home-based care. Home-based care is generally the best way of achieving good quality care and coverage in countries with strong family support and poor health infrastructure.

Countries with medium levels of resources should ensure that minimum standards for cancer pain relief and palliative care are progressively adopted at all levels of care, and that, nationwide, there is increasing coverage of patients through services provided by health care workers and home-based care.

Countries with high levels of resources should ensure that national pain relief and palliative care guidelines are adopted by all levels of care and that, nationwide, there is high coverage of patients through a variety of options, including home-based care.

CANCER CONTROL RESEARCH

8

The goal of cancer control research is to identify and evaluate means of reducing cancer morbidity and mortality, as well as of improving the quality of life of cancer patients and their families. Research is thus a key component in the development, implementation and evaluation of a national cancer control programme, which needs to have a scientific basis for identifying the causes of cancer, and for effective strategies for the prevention, treatment, and control of cancer, as well as for evaluating overall programme performance.

DEVELOPMENT OF NATIONAL CAPACITY FOR CANCER RESEARCH

The *Report on Health Research 2000* defines research capacity development as "a process in which individuals, organizations and societies develop abilities (individually and collectively) to perform functions effectively, efficiently and in a sustainable manner that respond to key questions on the major needs of the country and the entire population. This implies research capacity development is an ongoing learning and teaching process that involves individual researchers, their institutional environment, the policy makers and the people who will ultimately benefit from it" (Global Forum for Health Research, 2000).

The planning of a general research strategy and the setting of research priorities should be a continuous activity within a national cancer control programme. The planning, monitoring, and evaluation processes are critical not only for implementing the national programme, but also for the identification of gaps in available knowledge. The availability of national mechanisms to make objective decisions regarding the allocation of research resources and react rapidly to emerging problems and opportunities is of particular importance.

Research should be sensitive to local cultural norms and its focus should be specific to the country concerned (see Box 8.1). It should be linked as closely as possible to the most important cancer problems, to existing health services research, and to financial and other resources that will influence the scope of national cancer control efforts. Thus in one country, the most urgent problem may be one of maximizing the effectiveness of cervical screening programmes, while taking account of available treatment resources. For another country, the highest priority may be evaluation of approaches to providing palliative care services to all individuals with advanced disease.

Cancer control research is an important component of a national cancer control programme, but it should be carried out in collaboration with other programmes, rather than duplicating their work. This is particularly important in cancer prevention, as many components of cancer prevention are common to other chronic (noncommunicable) diseases. Moreover, cancer control research should be designed to provide information that can be shared with other disease control programmes.

RESEARCH AIMS

The three general research aims of cancer control research are fundamental research, translational research, and applications research (National Cancer Institute, (U.S.) 2002). Fundamental research aims to reduce the gap between ignorance and knowledge about cancer. While there has been dramatic progress in understanding the biological mechanisms underlying this disease and the development of effective treatment strategies, it is clear that many complex questions remain. *Translational research* aims to reduce the gap between knowledge and the translation of that knowledge into actions that can reduce morbidity and mortality from cancer. A solid base of scientific knowledge permits the rational development of prevention and

---

Box 8.1 **Criteria for setting priorities in national cancer control research**

The criteria for establishing priorities in cancer control research include the following elements:

- magnitude of cancer problem;
- expected cost-effectiveness of the intervention researched;
- effect on equity;
- probability of finding the solution;
- scientific quality of the research proposed;
- feasibility of the research proposed;
- ethical acceptability.

Adapted from: Global Forum for Health Research (2000) Global Forum for Health Research: An overview. Geneva, WHO.

treatment strategies, rather than a trial and error approach. *Applications research* aims to reduce the gap between what looks promising and what really works. Clinical trials and other field studies attempt to establish or refute the real benefit of new approaches to preventing or treating cancer, or to refute spurious claims. Programme evaluation is another form of applied research.

MAJOR AREAS OF RESEARCH

Research in cancer occurs in a wide range of scientific fields. The major categories of research are:
– laboratory;
– epidemiological;
– clinical;
– psychosocial and behavioural;
– health systems and health policies.

Most laboratory research is currently conducted in industrialized countries. It focuses on the elucidation of the biological mechanisms underlying cancer. Recent investigations of genetic and molecular/biological processes have produced dramatic and very promising results. Despite this, the causes underlying some of the most common cancer types are not yet well understood.

Epidemiology helps to identify environmental or human behavioural factors associated with cancer, even if the underlying mechanism is not clear, thus enabling decision-makers to implement effective intervention policies. The International Agency for Research on Cancer (IARC) in Lyon, France, is part of WHO and plays a fundamental role worldwide in cancer epidemiology.

Clinical trials are the basis for identification of promising therapies and determination of the most effective therapeutic strategies. The vast majority of clinical trials occur in developed countries and these account for the largest share of research resources. They serve as the basis for the licensing of drugs and other interventions, as well as the determination of optimal therapies to be included in national treatment guidelines. Trials for the prevention and early detection of cancer are often categorized as clinical research because of their nature and the similarity of research methodology to that of clinical trials.

Psychosocial and behavioural research also play an important role in cancer control. Scientific evidence to date indicates that thoughts and behaviour can have a significant impact on cancer onset and course, and vice versa. A major proportion of cancer in the world today is associated with lifestyles, such as the use of tobacco and alcohol, unhealthy diet, physical inactivity, and obesity. Psychosocial aspects also influence adherence to screening programmes or treatment modalities. The diagnosis and treatment of cancer are considerable sources of stress to patients, their families and health care providers, and this has a socioeconomic impact of great relevance to the effectiveness of cancer control programmes.

Research on cancer policies and health systems is needed to establish evidence-based priorities and determine how preventive, treatment and palliative care services can best be implemented and organized in order to achieve effectiveness, efficiency and equity of access.

As in other fields, cancer research involves the use of multi-disciplinary teams. For example, programmes for the prevention of tobacco-associated cancers involve active collaboration among clinicians, educators, legislators, behavioural scientists, economists, and agronomists. A randomized clinical trial brings together the skills of clinicians, nurses, laboratory scientists, ethicists, regulatory specialists, biostatisticians, computer scientists, and professional data managers.

PHASES OF RESEARCH

The classification of cancer control research by phase is illustrated in Figure 8.1. This classification system presents a stepwise structure that is useful for both research planning as well as determining the level of reliability of the supporting scientific evidence for a cancer control strategy.

Figure 8.1
Classification of
cancer control
research by phase

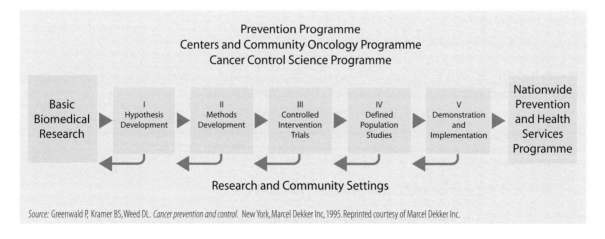

Source: Greenwald P, Kramer BS, Weed DL. *Cancer prevention and control.* New York, Marcel Dekker Inc, 1995. Reprinted courtesy of Marcel Dekker Inc.

Hypothesis development (phase I)

Investigations to develop hypotheses include observational epidemiological studies, such as case control studies associating specific types of cancer with previous dietary habits. A particularly useful type of phase I epidemiological investigation is a migrant study that involves comparisons of individuals of different origin living in the same place for different lengths of time. Such studies help define the relative importance of genetic and environmental factors in cancer causation and indicate the potential preventability of different cancers by showing the effect that a change in environment may have on the risk.

Methods development (phase II)

Studies to develop methods build upon the results of a hypothesis development investigation. They determine the feasibility of a specific intervention and gather preliminary information on whether the benefits of the intervention outweigh the risks involved. For example, a recent phase II study demonstrated the practicality of the early detection of asymptomatic cases of early cervical cancer by visual inspection with acetic acid (VIA) (Sankaranarayanan et al, 1997). The potential benefit of this low cost approach in developing countries is substantial, not only because it reduces the need for cytology screening laboratories, but because it also provides an immediate result, thereby avoiding the necessity of a patient tracking and recall system.

Controlled intervention trials (phase III)

A key phase in research is the controlled intervention trial. Such studies are frequently designed to compare a new intervention with the current standard intervention, using randomization to establish comparable patient groups for scientific comparison. Often involving hundreds of subjects, these studies are designed according to stringent scientific principles to provide a definitive answer to the extent of benefit, or lack thereof, that a new intervention offers. For example, a phase III randomized investigation comparing two groups of about 30 000 women demonstrated a 30% reduction in breast cancer mortality associated with mammography screening and clinical examination for women more than 50 years of age (Shapiro, 1997).

Defined population studies (phase IV)

A defined population study should be done after an intervention has been shown to be effective in a controlled comparison study. In a controlled comparison (phase III) study, the subjects are usually very motivated and the research environment is highly structured. A defined population study (phase IV) typically evaluates mechanisms to implement the intervention in a realistic general population situation, such as a city, state or region, and includes the generation of information on practical programme implementation and cost-effectiveness. For example, a defined population (phase IV) study of the prevention of cancer by smoking cessation would involve public education methods to encourage heavy smokers to join smoking cessation groups, conducting group programmes for smoking cessation, and individual counselling approaches.

Demonstration and implementation (phase V)

Ideally, national programme implementation should occur only after an intervention has successfully passed through each of the first four phases. The earlier phase III study should have provided clear scientific evidence demonstrating the extent of benefit of the intervention, and the phase IV study should have provided information about the practical implementation of the programme in a typical geographic region.

An understanding of these five phases of research can help determine the level of evidence that is available to support a cancer control intervention. The phase of research that has been completed indicates the strength of the scientific evidence available. For example, national cytology-based cervical cancer screening programmes in some Scandinavian countries have demonstrated a substantial national level decrease in the incidence of invasive cervical cancer. These results constitute phase V level information. The promising VIA approach to cervical cancer screening has successfully passed phase II, but still requires comparison (phase III) and defined population (phase IV) investigations before national level implementation should be considered. It is sometimes not possible to carry out all phases of cancer control research before promoting a cancer control intervention. For example, so far there has been no successful Phase III trial that has demonstrated the efficacy of cessation of tobacco smoking in the prevention of lung cancer, nor of cytology screening in preventing the development of invasive cancer of the cervix. Yet both these interventions have been successful in cancer control, as shown by evaluation of Phase V applications in several populations. Similarly, it seems unlikely, given the time that would be required, that there will ever be a Phase III trial that shows that dietary modification reduces the incidence of colorectal cancer. Yet colorectal cancer incidence and mortality are falling in North America, probably at least in part because of dietary modification, primarily introduced to control cardiovascular disease. Therefore, cancer control measures have to be introduced with regard to their likely efficacy and safety, and then evaluated carefully in the population to ensure they do in fact result in the expected impact, as discussed further in Chapter 12.

ease. Therefore, cancer control measures have to be introduced with regard to their likely efficacy and safety, and then evaluated carefully in the population to ensure they do in fact result in the expected impact, as discussed further in Chapter 12.

PROMOTING EVIDENCE-BASED CANCER CONTROL

Evidence-based cancer control means that the policies and practices employed in the prevention, early detection and treatment of cancer are based on principles that have been proven through appropriate scientific methods. For example, clinical treatment decisions should be based on the published reports of phase III randomized clinical trials. If more than one or two clinical trials have evaluated a specific therapeutic strategy decision, a systematic analytic mechanism—the meta-analysis—can be used to synthesize the available information. However, as with other analytic tools, care needs to be taken that such evaluations are undertaken meticulously using objective methodology.

Evidence-based medicine is the systematic, scientific and explicit use of current best evidence in making decisions about the care of individual patients. It is based on the assumption that clinical experience is crucial, but that systematic observations are necessary in order to summarize evidence. Knowledge of the basic mechanisms of the disease is also necessary, but is an insufficient guide for selecting treatments for clinical practice. An understanding of certain rules of evidence is necessary in order to interpret the literature correctly. With hundreds of medical journals worldwide, the number of published studies is increasing at a rapid rate. But the quality of published investigations continues to vary widely, and clinicians need training in how to identify reliable studies and evaluate their results.

Evidence-based medicine has evolved to include both clinical practice and health care for populations. Evidence-based healthcare (Gray, 2001) provides health managers and policy makers with the best evidence available about the financing, organization and management of healthcare.

RESEARCH IN DEVELOPING COUNTRIES

Research studies to determine the most cost-effective cancer control strategies are especially relevant in developing countries, perhaps even more so than in industrialized countries. When the available resources are extremely limited, there is no room for inefficient approaches or misuse of available funds.

The range of disease control strategies is often very restricted in developing countries. Expensive drugs, complex treatment strategies, costly diagnostic equipment and nurse-intensive approaches are not feasible. Nevertheless, an active research programme can determine the optimal use of the limited local resources. National capacity development for cancer research should be especially encouraged in less developed countries, to allow such countries to deal effectively and efficiently with their own cancer problems through evidence-based decision-making.

PRIORITIES FOR GLOBAL CANCER RESEARCH

While it is not feasible to list here all the areas of cancer control research that should be pursued, the following areas hold particular promise for the control of the most common cancers worldwide.

Policy research

There is a global need, especially in the less developed world, to promote and support the development of *evidence-based discipline* in policy development—which is the systematic, scientific and explicit use of current best evidence in making decisions about intervention strategies. Evidence-based cancer control guarantees that policies and practices employed in the prevention, early detection and treatment of cancer are based on principles that have been proven through appropriate scientific methods. For example, clinical treatment decisions should be based on the published reports of phase III randomized clinical trials, and screening for cervical cancer should rely on phase IV studies. If more than one or two of such studies have evaluated a specific intervention strategy, a systematic analytic mechanism—the meta-analysis—can be used to synthesize the available information. *Cost-effectiveness analyses* are also key studies that should be fostered, especially in less developed counties, to support effective policy development in cancer control. They are a useful in assisting policy makers and programme managers to decide between different ways of spending their limited resources to reduce the cancer burden. These studies generally compare new interventions to current practice. Realistically, it is not possible for studies to be undertaken on every possible intervention in every country. Therefore, it is necessary to investigate ways in which the results of studies can be adapted or applied to different settings.

Programme implementation

Research to evaluate innovative methodologies for implementing evidence-based cancer control strategies in less developed countries should be encouraged. This may lead to models that can be adapted to similar settings. Evaluation of the performance of existing cancer control programmes using the quality dimensions of performance of health services (described in Chapter 12) is key to making progress in cancer control and achieving effectiveness and efficiency.

Psychosocial and behavioural research

Research on optimizing behaviour to achieve healthy lifestyles, as well as studies about psychosocial aspects that influence adherence to early detection programmes and long-term treatment, are greatly needed, especially in developing countries. Further research is required to elucidate whether psychosocial factors, through a direct influence on the physiological system, for example, through neuroendocrine and immune functioning, have a meaningful influence on the onset or course of cancer (Epping-Jordan, 1999).

Tobacco eradication

Tobacco elimination would dramatically reduce the number of cancer deaths, especially cancers of the lung and oral cavity, as well as deaths from cardiovascular disease and other chronic diseases. Research to determine the most effective way to significantly reduce tobacco use in populations should have the highest priority. A multi-factor approach is clearly needed, as the range of interventions includes public information, childhood education, modification of individual behaviour, modification of governmental and nongovernmental organization behaviour (for those that rely upon tobacco taxes, promotion and sale), agriculture (crop alternatives), and legislation. But perhaps the most important of all is the development of effective education strategies to ensure that young people do not initiate a tobacco habit, an area in which efforts to date have largely been ineffective (Tubiana, 1999).

Identification of effective strategies for prevention

The use of infant vaccines to prevent disease is a well-established and cost-effective global strategy. While the potential now exists to prevent a substantial number of liver cancers by infant vaccination with hepatitis B vaccine, major efforts should be made to extend this prevention strategy to other cancers. Of particular interest would be the development of low-cost effective human papillomavirus vaccines for the prevention of cervical cancer, *Helicobacter pylori* vaccines for the prevention of stomach cancer, and

Epstein–Barr virus vaccines for the prevention of lymphoma and cancer of the nasopharynx.

While the link between diet and cancer has been clearly demonstrated, few specific dietary determinants of cancer risk have been established. Large-scale, controlled investigations comparing various dietary strategies need to be conducted in order to determine the health benefits of specific healthy diet recommendations.

Early detection of breast and cervical cancer

Currently, effective screening programmes for breast cancer using mammography are only feasible in the few most highly industrialized countries, because of the considerable expense involved. Recent reviews of previously conducted controlled investigations have raised doubts regarding the overall effectiveness of mammography screening. Additional controlled investigations are needed, not only to settle the issue regarding the role of mammography, but also for the majority of the world's women to establish the extent of benefit, if any, that would be seen with breast cancer screening using clinician examination, breast self-examination, or other approaches.

Although cytology screening programmes for the early detection of cervical cancer can currently be recommended for developed countries and middle-income countries, cervical cancer is also a major health problem for women in the least developed countries, where cytology screening would place too many demands on available resources. Effective low-cost screening strategies appropriate for all resource settings need to be investigated. Of particular promise for cervical cancer is visual inspection with acetic acid (VIA). This low-technology approach has successfully demonstrated feasibility and is currently being investigated for effectiveness.

Widely applicable curative treatments for cancer

There has been a steady stream of advances in the treatment of many forms of cancer. The general trend has, however, also been an increasing complexity in diagnostic and therapeutic techniques. Some of the more recent treatments can only be administered at specialized cancer treatment centres in the industrialized countries. Some therapies can only be given at few, if any, hospitals in developing countries, and often not even in general hospitals in industrialized countries. As a result, the vast majority of cancer patients in the world are unable to benefit from the available cancer treatment. These realities should be kept in mind when designing, and choosing to fund, such trials. Those responsible for cancer control programmes should strongly encourage the development of trials that test technologies and applications that could be feasibly implemented in a variety of settings, including less developed countries.

Development of effective palliative care delivery models

WHO has developed effective, low-cost strategies for the relief of pain and palliative care. However, effective approaches for bringing these benefits to patients in the community have not yet been developed for many settings. Various models for the delivery of palliative care, especially for the patient at home, need to be developed and investigated. Effective palliative care models would not only benefit patients with cancer, but also patients with HIV/AIDS and other diseases.

SURVEILLANCE IN CANCER CONTROL

9

Surveillance is the continuous collection of data for public health decision-making. In the context of a national cancer control programme, a surveillance programme should provide data on a continuing basis on incidence, prevalence, mortality, diagnostic methods, stage distribution, treatment patterns, and survival. It can also provide information about important risk factors and the prevalence of exposure to those factors in the population. Surveillance, therefore, plays a crucial role in formulating the cancer control plan, as well as in monitoring its success. An effective surveillance system requires substantial and continuous effort. Benefit comes only from careful analysis of the collected data, and it is therefore essential to allocate adequate resources for that purpose when a surveillance system is planned.

A comprehensive national cancer control programme requires a system of surveillance of cancer, its determinants, and outcomes. Over the past 50 years, the concept of cancer surveillance has evolved, centred upon the population-based cancer registry as a core component of the cancer control strategy (Greenwald, Sondik, Young, 1986; Armstrong, 1992). The roles of cancer surveillance are:

- to assess the current magnitude of the cancer burden and its likely future evolution;
- to provide a basis for research on cancer causes and prevention;
- to provide information on prevalence and trends in risk factors;
- to monitor the effects of prevention, early detection/screening, treatment, and palliative care.

MEASURING THE BURDEN OF CANCER

Various statistics are available for assessing the burden of cancer, and of different types of cancer, in the population.

Incidence

Incidence of disease is clearly an important measure of burden, since it describes the new cases that will require medical attention. It is the key

105

measure when considering prevention. Measurement of incidence requires the identification of all new cases of disease in a defined population through some kind of case-finding mechanism, with record-linkage to ensure that persons are not confused with events. This is the function of the population-based cancer registry. Cancer registries may present incidence according to histological subtype of cancer, or stage of disease at diagnosis.

Mortality

Mortality rates have been more widely used, since these have been available for a much longer period, and usually for large (national) populations. They are used in evaluations comparing disease rates between different populations, and over time to study differences in disease risk. They also provide a measure of disease outcome for evaluating, for example, the effectiveness of programmes of prevention, early detection and treatment of cancer.

Person-years of life lost

The concept of person-years of life lost (PYLLs) refines traditional mortality rates by providing a weighting for deaths at different ages. This measure is widely used in health services planning. This approach has been taken a step further, with the development of indices such as quality-adjusted life years (QALYs) and disability-adjusted life years (DALYs). Essentially, these quantify the spectrum of morbidity in terms of its duration and severity between onset of a disease and death or recovery.

Survival

Survival from cancer is the measure most often used to evaluate cancer treatment. Computation of survival depends upon follow-up of diagnosed cancer patients, and the calculation of the proportion surviving after different intervals of time. Stage of disease is one of the most important determinants of survival. Overall survival in the population reflects many factors—the stage of disease (influenced by early diagnosis or screening) and the availability of, access to, and effectiveness of treatment. Stage-specific survival provides a more relevant indicator of effectiveness of therapy (although accuracy with which stage of disease is measured varies between populations, and over time).

Prevalence

Prevalence of cancer is a measure of cancer burden (Hakama et al., 1975) indicating the number of patients alive who require medical care. However, there is no standard definition of a prevalent case of cancer. In theory, it should refer to someone once diagnosed as having cancer who is still alive; but this includes long survivors who are 'cured', and scarcely relates to 'burden', if the latter is being used to determine resource allocations. A reasonable compromise is to regard only patients alive between 0 and 5 years after diagnosis as 'prevalent' cancers, since this approximates the period of active treatment and follow-up of cases. Prevalence can be estimated directly by some cancer registries from their files of registered cases who have not died. Alternatively, prevalence can be estimated from the incidence of disease and survival curves, either for short-term survivors (for example, up to 5 or 10 years) or, if incidence and survival data are available for long periods, including long-term survivors also.

POPULATION-BASED CANCER REGISTRY

Disease registers are part of the surveillance system for several diseases, but they have been more important, and successful, for cancer than for any other condition. This is because of the serious nature of most cancers, which means that, except in a few societies without access to medical care, patients will almost always present for diagnosis and treatment. This has permitted the development and use of cancer registries, particularly population-based registries, which relate the incident cancer cases to a defined population-at-risk (Jensen et al., 1991).

The population-based cancer registry collects data on every person with cancer in a defined population, usually comprising people resident in a well-defined geographical region. The cooperation of the medical profession and health care services is vital to the success of cancer registration. The population-based cancer registry provides incidence rates, and the emphasis is on epidemiology and public health.

A major source of information and advice about population-based cancer registries and international data from such registries is the International Agency for Research on Cancer (IARC), a part of WHO. Located in Lyon, France, IARC should be called upon to assist in any planned development or reorganization of a cancer registry.

The emphasis of a cancer registry should be on the quality of the data collected, rather than on the quantity. Some of the most successful and productive registries collect only a very limited amount of data for each patient. Registries in developing countries should collect only the basic information common to all registries. This includes subject identification (including age and sex), ethnicity, incidence date, site and histology of the tumour, and the most valid basis of diagnosis. Other items, which are extremely useful, include the extent of disease (stage) and disease outcome for survival.

The establishment of a population-based cancer registry is highly desirable in the development of a national cancer control programme. Such registries are useful in the context of documenting the cancer patterns in a given region/country, in measuring cancer burden and in studying survival from cancer as well as in evaluating trends in the incidence of cancers over time. Thus they are valuable for the evaluation of national cancer control programmes. Hospital-based information systems provide valuable sources of information regarding methods of diagnosis, stage distribution, treatment methods, response to treatment, and survival, although accurate information on cancer incidence is unobtainable because of case referral and population coverage issues.

STATISTICS ON CANCER MORTALITY

Information on deaths from cancer in the population is collected by civil registration systems recording vital events (births, marriages, deaths). The responsible authority varies between countries, but usually the first level of data collection and processing is the municipality or province, with collation of national statistics being the responsibility of the Ministry of Health, or Ministry of the Interior. Mortality data are derived from death certificates on which information about the person dying and the cause of death is certified, usually by a medical practitioner. The International Classification of Diseases (ICD) (WHO, 1992) provides a uniform system of nomenclature and coding, and a recommended format for the death certificate. Mortality statistics are produced according to the underlying cause of death, which may not necessarily equate with the presence of a particular tumour.

About two-fifths of the world population is covered by national vital registration systems producing mortality statistics on cancer. This includes all of the developed countries, but only some developing countries. Even when national statistics are published, their quality is not the same in all countries. In some, coverage of the population is incomplete, and the mortality rates produced are implausibly low. In others, quality of cause of death information is poor.

THE WHO STEPWISE APPROACH FOR
MEASURING KEY RISK FACTORS

The WHO stepwise approach to surveillance (STEPS) is the WHO-recommended surveillance tool for measuring key risk factors for noncommunicable diseases. WHO is building one common approach to defining core variables for surveys, surveillance and monitoring instruments. The goal is to achieve data comparability over time and between countries. STEPS offers an entry point for low-income and middle-income countries to get started in the prevention of noncommunicable disease. It is a simplified approach providing standardized materials and methods as part of technical collaboration with countries, especially those that lack resources.

Because many factors associated with disease cannot be modified, emphasis in any surveillance system should be on those risk factors that are amenable to intervention. Surveillance of just seven selected risk factors (see Table 9.1) that reflect a large part of the future burden of noncommunicable diseases can provide a measure of the success of interventions.

The rationale for selecting these core risk factors is that: they have the greatest impact on the mortality and morbidity associated with noncommunicable diseases; modification is possible through effective primary prevention; measurement of these risk factors has been proven to be feasible and reliable; and measurements can be obtained using acceptable standard methodologies.

The stepwise approach encourages the development of an increasingly comprehensive and complex surveillance system depending on local needs (see Figure 9.1). Countries take the first step by adopting standardized questionnaires and adding modules, as appropriate, regarding behaviours such as tobacco and alcohol use. Questions that form the core data for each of these areas are simple and few in number and assure international comparability. Once the first step is in place, countries can build upon it by providing physical measurements in the second step. The third step involves

Table 9.1
Risk factors common to major noncommunicable diseases

Risk factor	Cancer	Cardiovascular disease[1]	Diabetes	Respiratory diseases[2]
Tobacco use	✓	✓	✓	✓
Alcohol	✓	✓		
Unhealthy diet	✓	✓	✓	✓
Physical inactivity	✓	✓	✓	✓
Obesity	✓	✓	✓	✓
Raised blood pressure		✓		

1 Including heart disease, stroke, and hypertension
2 Including chronic-obstructive pulmonary disease and asthma

the collection of biochemical measurements, most often by blood samples. At each step there is a core of information for each risk factor, an expanded core, and optional information, with the information of greater complexity being added sequentially as resources allow. WHO emphasizes that for surveillance to be sustainable, small amounts of good quality data are more valuable than large amounts of poor quality data.

At the country level, the implementation of this stepwise approach provides basic strategic public health information that can serve as the basis for planning and monitoring national prevention programmes as well as serving as an international standard for comparison purposes. The stepwise sequential process builds national capacity in a manner that is sustainable for the implementation of effective disease prevention programmes.

SURVEILLANCE INFRASTRUCTURE

Establishment of an effective surveillance system depends upon a continuing commitment of resources, including personnel and technology, for communication, data collection and analysis. A central or lead agency should be identified to coordinate the surveillance activities and produce a periodic overall surveillance report. A partnership approach should be used that includes receiving input from all participating agencies, collaboratively planning surveillance activities and the expansion of those activities, jointly interpreting the surveillance data, and jointly evaluating the performance and weaknesses of the surveillance system. The partners, whether at the national or local level, will thus share ownership of the system and the surveillance information produced.

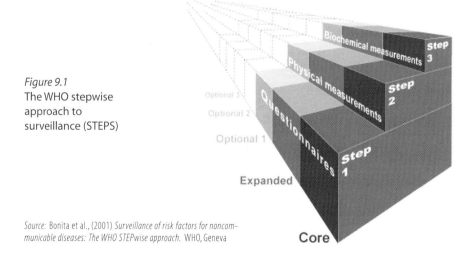

Figure 9.1
The WHO stepwise
approach to
surveillance (STEPS)

Source: Bonita et al., (2001) *Surveillance of risk factors for noncommunicable diseases: The WHO STEPwise approach.* WHO, Geneva

Managing a National Cancer Control Programme

There is little evidence so far of a balanced use of resources for population-wide control of cancer by governmental and nongovernmental bodies acting in partnership. Yet the evidence exists that would allow us to prevent at least one-third of the 10 million cancer cases that occur annually throughout the world. Current knowledge would also allow the early detection and effective treatment of a further one-third of those cases. Pain relief and palliative care can also improve the quality of life of patients and their families. With competent management that includes careful planning, implementation, monitoring and evaluation, the establishment of national cancer control programmes offers the most rational means of achieving a substantial degree of cancer control, even where resources are severely limited. It is for this reason that the establishment of a national cancer control programme is recommended wherever the burden of the disease is significant, there is a rising trend of cancer risk factors and there is a need to make the most efficient use of limited resources.

Planning a national cancer control programme means assessing strategic options and choosing those that are feasible, effective, and cost-effective, bearing in mind the specific conditions of the country concerned (Chapter 10).

Implementing a programme requires resources and processes, all of which have to be well managed. This issue is discussed in Chapter 11, along with the range of global initiatives that national cancer control programmes can draw on for experience and support. Moreover, in order to ensure that activities contribute to achieving the priorities that have been established, the programme will also need to be monitored and evaluated (Chapter 12).

PLANNING A NATIONAL CANCER CONTROL PROGRAMME

10

WHAT IS A NATIONAL CANCER CONTROL PROGRAMME?

A national cancer control programme is a public health programme designed to reduce the incidence and mortality of cancer and improve the quality of life of cancer patients in a particular country or state, through the systematic and equitable implementation of evidence-based strategies for prevention, early detection, treatment, and palliation, making the best use of available resources.

The following list summarizes the principles essential to a national cancer control programme based on quality management (ISO, 1997):

- *goal orientation* that continuously guides the processes towards improving the health and quality of life of the people covered by the programme;
- *focused on the needs of the people*, which implies focusing on the target population while addressing the needs of all stakeholders and ensuring their active involvement;
- *systematic decision-making process*, based on evidence, social values, and efficient use of resources, that benefits the majority of the target population;
- *systemic and comprehensive approach*, meaning that the programme is a comprehensive system with interrelated key components at the different levels of care, sharing the same goal, integrated with other programmes, to the health system and tailored to the social context (Figure 10.1), rather than a vertical programme operating in isolation;
- *leadership* that creates clarity and unity of purpose, and that encourages team building, broad participation, ownership of the process, continuous learning, and mutual recognition of efforts made;
- *partnership*, enhancing effectiveness through mutually beneficial relationships, built on trust and complementary capacities, with partners from different disciplines and sectors,

Figure 10.1
National cancer control programme: a systemic and comprehensive approach

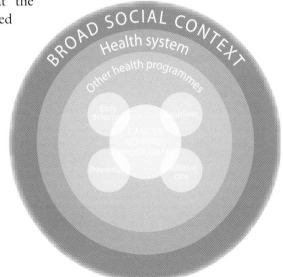

113

- *continuous improvement, innovation and creativity* to maximize performance, and to address social and cultural diversity, and the new needs and challenges presented by a changing environment.

WHY ESTABLISH A NATIONAL CANCER CONTROL PROGRAMME?

Previous chapters of this monograph have provided the scientific background to current knowledge of the causes of cancer, and the components of cancer control: prevention, early detection, treatment and palliative care, cancer control research, and cancer surveillance. With careful planning and appropriate priorities, the establishment of a national cancer control programme offers the most rational means of achieving a substantial degree of cancer control, even where resources are severely limited. For this reason, the establishment of a national cancer control programme is recommended wherever the burden of the disease is significant, there is a rising trend of cancer risk factors, and there is a need to make the most efficient use of limited resources.

Without careful planning, there is a risk that the resources available for cancer control will be used inefficiently, and that the benefits to the population that should flow from the use of such resources will not be realized. In the absence of any national coordinating mechanism, it is possible that limited resources will largely be consumed for the treatment of cancer by prestigious hospitals. Such institutions often serve only selected sub-populations and may do little to reduce the national cancer burden. In contrast, an effective cancer control programme comprises an integrated set of activities covering all aspects of cancer prevention and control, and it operates with an appropriate allocation of available resources among the various activities and equitable coverage of the population.

WHICH COUNTRIES HAVE NATIONAL CANCER CONTROL PROGRAMMES?

A WHO survey of 167 countries in 2001 assessed national capacity for prevention and control of cancer, as well as of other noncommunicable diseases (WHO, 2001b). The results of this survey (see Table 10.1) show that nearly half of the 167 countries responding indicated that they had a cancer control policy or plan. About two-thirds of the countries indicated the availability of national guidelines for prevention, and almost half specified that cancer management guidelines had been produced. While objective data are difficult to obtain (two-thirds of the countries did not provide supporting documents confirming the existence of these plans and guidelines), this survey demonstrates an awareness in many countries of the need for the planning of programmes to prevent and control cancer.

According to the information collected for a WHO meeting in 2000 on national cancer control programmes, only a few countries have developed nationwide, comprehensive cancer control programmes that include prevention, early detection, treatment and palliative care. Various countries have developed important initiatives at the state or provincial level; others have focused on one or two priority areas, achieving national coverage in some cases.

The major elements of national cancer control programmes in the Americas and in the Western Pacific are described, respectively, in Tables 10.2 and 10.3, by way of example. In the Americas, comprehensive cancer control strategies that address the full spectrum of prevention, early detection, diagnosis, treatment and palliative care for one or more cancer sites exist in five countries: Brazil, Canada, Chile, Colombia and the United States. Most countries are involved in specific cancer efforts, which may not be comprehensive in nature, but that are designed to reduce risks and address some aspects of cancer control. In Latin America, palliative care services for people with advanced cancers are just beginning to be included as part of cancer care.

In the Western Pacific, cervical cancer screening, national tobacco control programmes and routine hepatitis B vaccination are among the activities

Table 10.1 National capacity for cancer prevention and control

Region	Number of countries responding (%)	Countries with cancer control policy or plan	Availability of national guidelines		Primary health care (anti-neoplastic drugs)	
			Prevention	Management	Availability	Affordability
Africa	39 (85%)	15%	29%	43%	22%	11%
The Americas	33 (95%)	50%	83%	48%	57%	30%
Eastern Mediterranean	17 (77%)	56%	60%	33%	77%	36%
Europe	41 (80%)	62%	84%	59%	91%	90%
South-East Asia	10 (100%)	78%	43%	43%	43%	17%
Western Pacific	27 (100%)	64%	65%	47%	74%	64%
Overall	167 (87%)	48%	67%	48%	60%	46%

Source: World Health Organization (2001b) Assessment of national capacity for noncommunicable disease prevention and control. The report of a global survey. Geneva, WHO.

115

implemented. Legislation to make morphine available has been passed in fewer than half of the countries, and the monitoring of progress in cancer control is routinely done in only four countries in this region.

The experience of the cancer control programme in Kerala, India, is described in Box 10.1.

Common hindrances to a national cancer control programme and benefits often seen after development of such a programme are summarized in Table 10.4.

Table 10.2 Cancer control in the Americas*
(Countries with a partial or comprehensive national cancer policy/strategy)

Country	Major elements of the strategy
Cuba	Breast cancer screening policy; cervical cancer programme
Ecuador	Cervical cancer programme; breast cancer screening policy
Peru	Cervical cancer programme
Venezuela	Cervical cancer plan; breast cancer policy
Mexico	Breast and cervical cancer programmes
Brazil	Comprehensive cancer control strategy
Panama	Breast cancer screening programme
Costa Rica	National cervical cancer programme
Colombia	Strategies for information systems, education, intersectoral coordination, research and legislation
Chile	Prevention, cervical and breast cancer programmes, curable tumours and palliative care
Barbados	Cervical cancer plan
Canada	Canadian Strategy for Cancer Control; Canadian Breast Cancer Initiative
USA	Targets: lung, breast, cervix, colorectal, oral, prostate and skin cancer

* Countries are listed in ascending order of their per capita health expenditure

Table 10.3. Cancer Control in the Western Pacific*
(Countries with a multi-sectoral policy for cancer control activities)

Country	Major elements of the strategy
Mongolia	Cervical cancer screening; tobacco control programme, cancer treatment guidelines; morphine available for cancer pain relief
Cambodia	Tobacco control programme
China	Cervical and breast cancer screening; cancer treatment guidelines
Niue	Cervical and breast cancer screening; tobacco control programme
Philippines	Cervical and breast cancer screening, tobacco control programme; cancer treatment guidelines; morphine available for cancer pain relief
Samoa	Cervical cancer screening; tobacco control programme
Malaysia	Cervical and breast cancer screening; tobacco control programme; cancer treatment guidelines
Fiji	Cervical cancer screening, cancer treatment guidelines and morphine available for cancer pain relief
Singapore	Tobacco control programme; cancer treatment guidelines; morphine available for cancer pain relief
Korea, Rep.	Cervical and breast cancer screening; tobacco control programme; cancer treatment guidelines; morphine available for cancer pain relief
New Zealand	Cervical and breast cancer screening; tobacco control programme; cancer treatment guidelines; morphine available for cancer pain relief
Australia	Cervical and breast cancer screening; tobacco control programme; cancer treatment guidelines; morphine available for cancer pain relief

* Countries are listed in ascending order of their per capita health expenditure

WHO SHOULD BE INVOLVED IN PLANNING A NATIONAL CANCER CONTROL PROGRAMME?

The motivation to initiate a national cancer control programme or improve the performance of an existing programme can come from different sectors within the country or can be a combined effort with international organizations. In close collaboration with its Member States and other partners, WHO has developed a global strategy for the prevention and control of noncommunicable diseases in which cancer control appears as one of the major priorities. WHO headquarters, regional and country offices can be

---

Box 10.1 The cancer control programme of Kerala, India

The national cancer control programme of India was formulated in 1984, focusing on: the primary prevention of tobacco-related cancers, as 50% of all cancer in India was due to tobacco use; early detection of cancers of accessible sites, as the three major forms of cancer were accessible; augmentation of treatment facilities; and establishment of equitable pain control and a palliative care network throughout the country, as more than 80% of cancer patients reported in very late stages.

In 1988, Kerala was the first state in India to formulate a cancer control programme (called a 10 year action plan), with the same goals as the national plan. Kerala is a state in southwest India with a population of 31 million. The well-integrated health service is provided by the government and the private sector. A hospital cancer registry, started in 1982, was a major source of information for planning the programme.

Tobacco habit prevention

Two state-wide programmes targeted teenagers, through the schools. In one programme, 126 000 families were declared "tobacco free". A second programme, using a similar approach, was implemented in over 6 000 schools.

Training regarding anti-tobacco messages was given to 5 000 doctors and over 9 000 other health workers. More than 130 000 volunteers were trained to support the anti-tobacco messages throughout the villages. Executive orders have banned smoking in educational institutions, government offices, public transport and other public places. A reduction in tobacco consumption of 1% per year has been seen in the Trivandrum Oral Cancer Screening project area.

Early detection programme

Because high technology methods were beyond reach, activities focused on education to improve awareness, followed by diagnosis and treatment. Screening camps were organized periodically, with the support of the government and voluntary organizations. Self-examination of the oral cavity, breast self-examination and physician breast-examination were taught; cytology-based screening for cervical cancer augmented this initiative. At the village level, 12 600 volunteers were trained to create awareness of early signs of cancer, and motivate people to undergo tests and therapy, if needed. The success of Kerala's programmes can be greatly attributed to the Early Cancer Detection Centres (ECDC), which serve as focal points for coordination of the early detection activities and the provision of clinical examination, cytology and histopa-

thology. Initially established as government programmes, two are now run by the Regional Cancer Centre and five by nongovernmental organizations. The public sees the role of ECDCs to be the screening of normal (asymptomatic) people, whereas hospitals are recognized as places for sickness management. The ECDC at Erankulam has screened more than 80 000 people since its inception in 1984.

Pain relief and palliative care

A pain control and palliative care division was started by the Regional Cancer Centre in 1986. In 1988 it was the first institution in India to manufacture and supply morphine liquid. Morphine tablets were first made available in 1991 and are now locally manufactured. A cancer pain relief network has been established, consisting of two nodes and 16 peripheral centres. A unit to make home visits to terminally ill patients and to train the relatives of these patients in principles of cancer pain control was initiated in 2000, and will be expanded.

Evaluation

This programme was found to achieve a reduction in tobacco consumption, down-staging of advanced tumours, augmentation of comprehensive therapy programmes, and a network of palliative care centres.

called upon to provide technical assistance and advice in support of the promotion of national cancer control programmes at the country or state level.

With appropriate mobilization of all the stakeholders, it is possible to develop cancer control policies that are acceptable to the people for whom they are intended, affordable, integrated with other national health programmes, and linked effectively with sectors other than health that are relevant to cancer control.

People involved in formulating and implementing the overall strategy for the national cancer control programme should be health professionals with experience in disease control and large-scale health programmes, cancer experts, other health service workers, patients' groups, and representatives from other sectors involved. Governmental and nongovernmental leaders in the cancer field need to work together closely to develop a successful programme. The national cancer control programme should involve the general public, whose knowledge and awareness of the problem can, and should, become a major force in combating cancer. As a significant and growing aspect of a nation's health problems, cancer requires the attention of the highest levels of government as well as community involvement.

Political commitment is essential. It should be the responsibility of health leaders to persuade political leaders, health practitioners, and the public as to the magnitude of the national cancer problem and inform them what can be done to overcome it. It is particularly important to emphasize the multifaceted nature of the problem, the essential role of prevention to reduce the future cancer burden, and the current role of early detection, as well as treatment and palliative care.

Table 10.4
Common
hindrances to
and benefits
from a national
cancer control
programme

Hindrances	Benefits
Low priority given to cancer by Ministry of Health	Promotes equal coverage of services (social justice)
Lack of public support	Raises political awareness of the issues
Shortage of resources	Better use of available funds, avoiding misuse
Excess reliance on treatment	Puts priorities into perspective, especially the role of prevention
Uncritical use of Western approach	Local technology can be used
Shortage of trained staff	Education of health professionals first
Cultural and religious factors	Programme development leading to process ownership
Lack of understanding by health professionals	Identifies scientific basis of activities
Limited access to oral morphine	Ethical obligation to relieve suffering at reasonable cost
Viewed as vertical programming	

HOW TO PLAN A NATIONAL
CANCER CONTROL PROGRAMME?

Ideally, the process of establishing a national cancer control programme should be organized, democratic, empowering, and pragmatic, with the boundaries of the programme defined by the social, medical, and political environment of the country concerned. In a national cancer control programme, there is a need to address managerial, technical and financial needs, with evidence-based policy development and involvement of all stakeholders. The aim should be balanced cancer control actions extending to the whole country in an equitable way. Although it is clear that objectives and priorities need to be tailored to the specific country context, the planning processes to be undertaken in all countries – whether a programme is to be introduced for the first time or an existing programme is to be revised to make it more effective – are sufficiently similar to allow for the use of models. Since the first edition of this WHO publication, various countries have developed frameworks for comprehensive cancer control programmes that add new value to the original model elaborated by WHO. An example of such a model is shown in Figure 10.2.

The following model is based on those experiences and comprises phases for planning and implementing a national cancer control programme. As in the model illustrated in Figure 10.2, the phases require the active participation of stakeholders, follow a circular path, and experience a continuous exchange of information for adequate decision making, thus allowing for sustained improvement and adjustment to new needs and knowledge.

The planning process is described below. Chapter 11 proceeds to deal with implementation, and Chapter 12 looks at monitoring and evaluation.

Assessing the magnitude of the cancer problem

As an initial step, a national cancer control programme requires an analysis of the cancer burden and risk factors in the target area, as well as a capacity assessment (analysis of existing facilities, programmes and services in the broader social context).
Four categories of information are needed for the initial analysis:
- demographic data;
- cancer and risk factor data;
- data on other diseases;
- capacity assessment.

Demographic data
Generally speaking, demographic data, with appropriate projections, are

fairly readily available through national censuses. Because cancer rates vary by age, sex and, in some countries, race, data on these population characteristics are essential.

Cancer data and cancer risk factor data

Epidemiological data on the occurrence of cancer, and knowledge of causative factors and of how to avoid those factors, provide a basis for determining where the emphasis of cancer control efforts should be placed. Details on the processes required for surveillance of cancer are provided in Chapter 9. A cancer surveillance programme, built around a population-based cancer registry, has a major role in providing the data to justify the establishment of a national cancer control programme, as well as in monitoring the progress of implementation of the cancer control programme.

For a comprehensive assessment of the cancer burden, it is desirable to have incidence, survival and mortality data for all forms of cancer combined, and for each of the most common forms of the disease. Other indicators of "burden", such as prevalence, (PYLL), (DALY), may also be calculated. Such information is essential for setting priorities for the national cancer control programme, including the planning of cancer-related health care services. If a population-based cancer registry does not exist, incidence will have to be estimated.

When incidence or mortality data are available for several years, an evaluation of time trends in cancer, and how these vary according to age group (or year of birth), sex, or other characteristics of the population, is possible. These data may be used to project the likely evolution of the cancer pattern in future years. The most important variables for forecasting the future burden are overall population trends, changes in the age structure of the population, and the prevalence of important risk factors, especially tobacco use 20–30 years earlier. In assessing the future cancer burden, potential changes in the relative importance of various cancers, the impact of cancer control measures, and forecasting of trends in incidence and mortality are valuable. Projections usually involve the assumption that past trends in rates of incidence or mortality will be maintained, and will apply to projected changes in the population. This assumption is often in error. Experience shows that, for many cancers, past trends will not be maintained because of changes in environmental risk factors, and the development of new techniques for prevention, early detection, and treatment. Projections nevertheless provide a useful benchmark against which the impact of all future changes, including the interventions of the national cancer control programme, can be evaluated.

Estimates of the numbers of cancer cases and deaths due to cancer may be higher than the numbers known to the health services. In countries where awareness of cancer is low and access to health care is limited, only a small proportion of actual cases are known to the health services. With greater awareness of cancer, a higher proportion of people with the disease will present to the health services for care. Thus, demands for care will rise more rapidly than the increase in need resulting from increased incidence.

Data on other diseases

It is essential to establish the importance of cancer relative to that of other diseases. Good vital-statistics systems will provide the necessary data on mortality but, in their absence, proxy data, such as hospital admissions by cause, may have to be used.

Figure 10.2
Framework for comprehensive cancer prevention and control

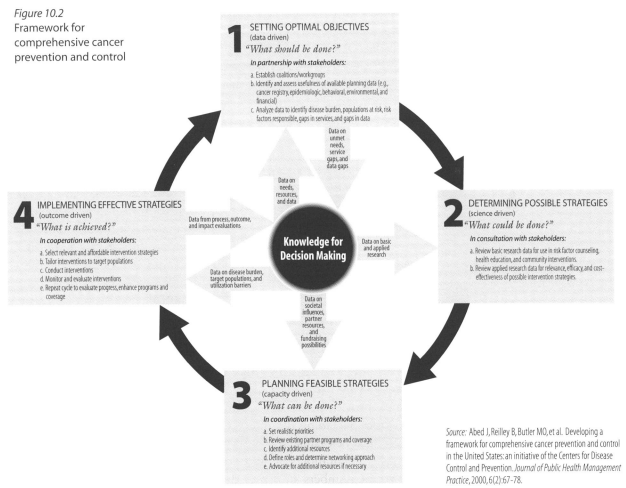

Source: Abed J, Reilley B, Butler MO, et al. Developing a framework for comprehensive cancer prevention and control in the United States: an initiative of the Centers for Disease Control and Prevention. *Journal of Public Health Management Practice*, 2000, 6(2):67-78.

The relative burden of cancer in the future is a function not only of the absolute amount of cancer, but also of trends in other causes of death. In most countries, a decrease in deaths from infectious diseases or cardiovascular disease is followed by an increase in the number of cancer deaths. The net result is that deaths from cancer will constitute an increasing proportion of all deaths.

Capacity assessment

According to the United Nations Development Programme, "capacity can be defined as the ability of individuals and organizations or organizational units to perform functions effectively, efficiently and sustainably in a given socio-political context". This definition implies that capacity is not a passive state but part of a continuing process and that individuals, both providers and beneficiaries, are central to capacity development. The overall context in which organizations function is also a key element. (United Nations Development Programme, 1998).

Capacity assessment in the area of cancer involves collecting and analysing data on:

- the *overall context*, implying an examination of the broad economic, social, cultural and political conditions that are directly or indirectly related to the development of a national cancer control programme;
- the policy, and institutional environment of the *existing health system*[1] that directly or indirectly relate to cancer:
- overall health system performance (WHO, 2001c), health policies, laws, regulations, financing, organization and management of services according to levels of care, definitions of responsibilities of the public and private sectors;
- existing programmes and services for cancer prevention, early detection, treatment and palliation, including their organization, facilities, personnel, drugs and technologies, budgeting, and information and evaluation systems;
- quality performance indicators, such as effectiveness, efficiency, appropriateness, accessibility, and sustainability, which measure the interaction between the system and beneficiaries of cancer prevention and control activities;
- existing education and continuous training programmes in the technical and management field;

---

1 According to *The World Health Report 2000*, a health system is defined as: all organizations, institutions, and resources devoted to the production of health actions. Health actions are defined as any efforts whether in personal health care, public health services, or through intersectoral initiatives, whose primary purpose is to improve health.

- linkages of cancer prevention and control activities with other programmes, both in the health sector and other sectors, and partnerships between governmental and nongovernmental organizations.

The capacity assessment can be done quite simply, or at a greater level of complexity, depending on practical constraints such as budget, time, and availability of information. Whatever the degree of complexity, it is important to maintain a systemic approach that focuses on how the problem being studied interacts with the other constituents of the system. Instead of isolating small components, the systemic approach expands its view to take into account a large number of interactions. For example, a cytology cervical screening programme cannot be viewed as an isolated project. It should be considered as a subsystem of a cancer early detection programme, with various interacting components (primary health care clinics, pathology, colposcopy, and so on). At the same time, interaction with other programmes or initiatives, such as reproductive health, breast cancer screening, and clinical preventive services at the primary level of health care is essential (see Figure 10.3).

After the above-mentioned data have been collected and reviewed, they must be analysed to identify needs and gaps in services, as well as gaps in data. This analysis should provide a solid basis for setting objectives for the national cancer control programme.

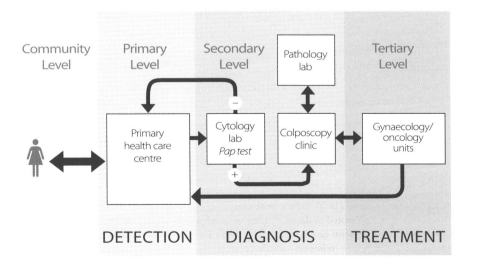

Figure 10.3
Example of programme processes in cervical cancer screening

Setting measurable cancer control objectives

A clear statement of aims, goals, and objectives is essential to any disease control strategy.

The overall aims of a national cancer control programme are to reduce the incidence and mortality of cancer, as well as to improve overall survival and the quality of life of cancer patients and their families.

The goals of a national cancer control programme may be summarized as follows:

– to prevent future cancers;
– to diagnose cancers early;
– to provide curative therapy;
– to ensure freedom from suffering;
– to reach all members of the population.

Objectives are more specific than general aims, and are formulated to achieve the goals. They cannot be fully specified in the absence of a detailed situation analysis or performance evaluation. Decisions on objectives for any particular country must "ensure that the limited resources are directed to areas of greatest need and support efforts with the highest probability of success" (Mertens, 1999). Cancer control objectives should be compatible with general health objectives and can be formulated along the lines of quality dimensions such as effectiveness, efficiency, and accessibility. Examples of possible objectives are listed below:

Reducing the risk of cancer:

• to reduce tobacco smoking rates among health care professionals and patients attending primary care clinics;
• to avoid passive smoking in the workplace, public transportation and public places;
• to increase physical activity and reduce overweight rates among young adults.

Detecting cancer earlier:

• to improve early diagnosis rates of cervical, breast, oral, colorectal, and skin cancers through raising awareness of early signs and symptoms;
• to develop an effective and efficient cytology screening programme for cervical cancer.

Provide curative therapy:

• to improve access to good quality, standardized treatments for all patients having early detectable cancers or cancers having high potential of curability;

- to ensure the use of non-invasive procedures for all patients with pre-cancerous cervical lesions.

End of life care:

- to improve control of symptoms and prolong physical autonomy in all patients with advanced cancer;
- to provide psychosocial assistance and facilitate spiritual support to the majority of incurable patients and their families.

Reduce inequalities:

- to ensure that prioritized cancer preventive and control services are provided to all sectors of the population.

Evaluating possible strategies for cancer control

The activities, standards and guidelines of a cancer strategy need to be based on sound and current scientific evidence. This requires expertise to critically review scientific information and evaluate the costs of various interventions. In particular, those designing the strategy need to understand how to analyse the evidence or undertake systematic reviews. If this expertise is not available within a country, outside experts should be called upon to assess the evidence. This assessment should highlight points for discussion and identify points of contention. For example, if there are conflicting research results, the original papers should be presented and the differences between them, including methodological differences, should be discussed.

Cost-effectiveness studies should be considered in the critical review. These usually consider only direct medical costs, an approach that works well in a public system with set pricing. It is, however, also important to assess cost-effectiveness based on societal perspectives, and to include non-medical as well as direct medical costs when evaluating strategies.

Further, the effectiveness of interventions needs to be defined as a function of tangible outcomes, based on epidemiological or clinical knowledge. The assumptions inherent in the stated outcomes need to be considered, especially as to whether or not they are applicable in a developing country.

Choosing priorities for initial cancer control activities

Once possible strategies are identified there is a need to choose those that are feasible to implement and that are acceptable and relevant to the society. In developed and developing countries alike, resources for cancer control (funds, trained people, equipment, and facilities) are insufficient to allow all possible activities to be undertaken. It is, therefore, essential that resources are used as effectively and efficiently as possible. Health authorities should, therefore, establish appropriate priorities.

When a range of possible activities has been identified, the measures of effectiveness and cost should be defined and the following steps carried out for each activity:

– identifying the immediate target;
– estimating the impact in terms of reduction in incidence or mortality;
– estimating the resources needed;
– estimating the cost of the activity.

A number of models have been developed by WHO and others to facilitate this process (Eddy, 1986; WHO, 1986a). It must be recognized, however, that the validity of a model is entirely dependent on the validity of the assumptions made and of the data entered into the model. The models incorporate epidemiological data, knowledge gained in research, and expert judgements for applying the principles of cost-effectiveness analysis in setting priorities. The use of such quantitative methods allows estimation of the impact of various cancer control activities in a population over a given period of time and thus permits priorities to be set.

The application of such methods in Chile in 1986, for example, indicated that, by 1995, the average cost of screening for cervical cancer beginning at age 35 years would be nearly a third less than the cost of screening starting at age 20 (Eddy, 1986). Either of these options, however, would be far more cost-effective than screening for stomach cancer, also a common cancer in Chile.

ASSESSMENT OF STRATEGIES FOR EIGHT COMMON CANCERS

Table 10.5 assesses the strategies for eight common cancers worldwide. In order to make the best use of resources, it is important to identify both effective strategies and strategies that are largely ineffective. Although it is difficult to place a cost on the various strategies for cancer control because of variations between countries, including different levels of existing infrastructure and differences in local strategy implementation, an approximate relative indicator of expense is also included in Table 10.5. In general, prevention and palliative care require less national resources commitment than early detection (screening) and treatment. However, the benefits of a cancer prevention programme will only be realized 20–30 years after effective implementation of the programme.

Since cancer control depends on the application of existing knowledge, no activity should be introduced unless its effectiveness is strongly supported by

Table 10.5 Assessment of strategies for eight common cancers

Site of cancer	Prevention		Early detection		Curative therapy		Palliative care	
Mouth/pharynx	++	$	−	$$	+	$$	++	$
Oesophagus	+	$	−		−		++	$
Stomach	++	$	+	$$	-		++	$
Colon/rectum	++	$	+	$$	+	$$	++	$
Liver	++	$	−		−		++	$
Lung	++	$	−		−		++	$
Breast	+	$	++	$	++	$	++	$
Cervix	+	$	++	$	++	$	++	$

++ effective; + partly effective; − largely ineffective
$ less expensive; $$ more expensive
Sources: Adapted from: Stjernswärd J. *Cancer control: Strategies and priorities. World Health Forum, 1985,* 6: 160–164

data from research programmes or from cancer control programmes elsewhere. Such programmes usually provide data that enable the costs of the activity to be estimated, although the information may have to be modified, for example, to reflect different salary scales, if it is to be relevant to another country. Once cost estimates have been made, it is possible to compare the effectiveness and cost of all activities, and make a rational decision about priorities for both current and proposed new activities. It is useful to classify priority areas in two groups: activities that can be introduced (or improved) without the need for additional resources, and activities that will require extra resources (staff, technology, drugs, and so on).

FORMULATING THE NATIONAL CANCER CONTROL PROGRAMME POLICY

Ideally, the national cancer control programme policy should be formulated once the planning process has been completed. It will provide a solid platform for implementing and maintaining the national cancer control programme.

A policy may be defined as an explicit commitment by government and its partners that provides objectives for a balanced cancer control programme, specifies the relative priority of each objective and indicates the resources and measures required to obtain the objectives. It should cover the following elements:

- the challenges posed by cancer, both now and in the future: current challenges are identified by the cancer data described above, together with information (if available) on the stage at diagnosis of the important cancers in the country;

Box 10.2 Cancer Policy as part of the National Health Plan

Fundamental, long-term social interests—including employment, productivity, and the economy, as well as health—can be served by making cancer control an integral part of a nation's health programme.

The WHO Seventh, Eighth, and Ninth General Programmes of Work for the periods 1984–1989, 1990–1995, and 1996–2001, respectively, all endorsed by the World Health Assembly, urge Member States to strengthen, or to consider initiating, the development of cancer control measures as an integral part of national health plans. Control of cancer can be achieved most efficiently in the context of a comprehensive national plan. A cancer control policy will enrich the total health effort, and cancer control efforts will themselves be enhanced by becoming an integral part of a total national health plan. Equity, within both oncology and other health services should be promoted.

Cancer prevention policy as a component of integrated health promotion and noncommunicable disease prevention policies

WHO has developed, in close collaboration with its Member States and other partners, a global strategy for the prevention and control of noncommunicable diseases in which cancer control appears as one of the four major priorities. The global strategy was endorsed by the 53rd World Health Assembly held in May 2000 and emphasizes the need for an integrated approach to health promotion and noncommunicable disease prevention strategies. Because tobacco use, alcohol, nutrition,

physical inactivity and obesity are risk factors common to other noncommunicable diseases, programmes to prevent cancer, cardiovascular disease, diabetes and respiratory diseases can effectively use the same surveillance and health promotion mechanisms. Close collaboration among the disease-specific stakeholders is necessary to maximize the effectiveness of the available resources and achieve the desired population behavioural changes. Regional networks are also recognized as an important approach to facilitate national programme development. The CINDI programme (Countrywide Integrated Noncommunicable Disease Intervention) in Europe and CARMEN programme in the Americas are regional networks. Both are repositories of a wealth of experience, especially regarding programme implementation.

Intersectoral aspects of a cancer control policy

Because the control of cancer involves so many social vectors—economic, educational and political—a broad, society-based approach is required; expertise in the disease alone will not suffice. The intersectoral approach requires analysis of all the social elements that can affect the control of cancer. Those concerned with cancer control must work with authorities in agriculture, commerce, communications, education, industry, and law in order to achieve success.

The spirit and philosophy of full participation must be part of the planning process. It is critical that the ministry of health understand, accept and adopt a stakeholder-driven

approach. The importance of involving a range of multiple stakeholders in the process must not be overlooked, since successful implementation depends on recommendations for the strategy originating from the groups that will eventually be expected to execute the strategy. Particularly important is ensuring the involvement of community representatives, notably cancer survivors who can offer insights into programme design based on their needs and experiences with the health care system. This is exemplified by the need to control tobacco use as a means of preventing cancer. Social and economic pressures are the key factors in the initiation and maintenance of tobacco addiction. Controlling tobacco use, therefore, requires a multisectoral and comprehensive approach. This may entail dealing with international agencies, governments, nongovernmental organizations, the media, the health professions, childhood education, as well as with civil society, to curb the tobacco epidemic. Another example is the need to increase the availability of oral morphine for palliative care, which requires the cooperation of drug regulators and legislators, in addition to the expertise of cancer specialists.

Intersectoral collaboration is also essential if programmes are to be cost-effective. The public cannot cope with conflicting educational messages coming from different sectors, such as one set of dietary recommendations for the avoidance of cancer and another for the avoidance of cardiovascular disease. Similar coordination is required for counselling on sexual lifestyles, designed to prevent sexually transmitted diseases, cervical cancer, and AIDS.

- the broad aims of the cancer control policy, which are:
  - prevention of cancer;
  - early detection, coupled with effective and efficient treatment of potentially curable disease;
  - relief of pain and palliative care to improve the quality of life of patients;
- the principles on which the policy is to be based;
- an explicit statement of goals, objectives and priorities within the policy;
- the programmes, both new and revised, that will be required to carry out the policy;
- the resources currently available and those that will be required to carry out the policy in full;
- the roles and responsibilities of those involved in carrying out the various activities at the different levels of the health system;
- any legislative measures that will be required, such as those to control tobacco use, allocate funds for recommended activities, or ensure the availability of oral morphine;
- indicators for monitoring and evaluating the national cancer control programme.

IMPLEMENTING A NATIONAL CANCER CONTROL PROGRAMME

11

MOVING FROM POLICY TO IMPLEMENTATION

The process of implementing a national cancer control programme needs competent management to identify priorities and resources (planning), and to organize and coordinate those resources to guarantee sustained progress to meet the planned objectives (implementation monitoring and evaluation). Good management is therefore essential to maintain momentum and introduce any necessary modifications. A quality management approach is essential to improving the performance of the programme. Such an approach encourages all participants in the programme, including staff volunteers, community groups, and patients to practice positive, initiative-taking behaviour and adopt a systematic approach to managing the various processes in order to prevent problems.

Schematically, the programme can be seen as a system, with inputs, processes, outputs, and outcomes (Figure 11.1). The inputs are the various resources needed to run the programme. The term resources is used here in a broad sense, implying people, staff, finance, facilities, techniques, methods, and so on. The processes are the means by which programme services are delivered, or how the programme organizes resources to carry out its mission. The outputs are the units of services provided or the direct products of programme activities. The outcomes are the impacts on the people receiving the services or participating in the programme.

What resources are needed for a national cancer control programme?

Leadership and team building

The various activities of a national cancer control programme share common objectives. Competent management is needed to integrate these activities into a coherent programme. Key to competent management is the leadership of the programme, who should be facilitative, participatory and empowering in how vision and goals are established and carried out. A coordinator and a board constitute the core of the programme management. Whenever possi-

131

ble, both should be appointed early in the establishment of a national cancer control programme and given appropriate responsibility and support.

Ideally, the individual selected as the programme coordinator should have technical competence and political influence, charisma, good management and communication skills, and relevant knowledge and experience in public health. It is also desirable for this individual to have expertise in public relations, fundraising, lobbying, consensus building, information systems and evaluation techniques. It may not be possible to find all these characteristics in one person, and a leadership team may therefore be a preferable solution. The coordinator needs to keep a balance among the prevention, treatment and palliative care components. This person also needs to be persevering, flexible and creative, in order to overcome the numerous barriers the programme will face.

In addition to organizing the work of the board, the coordinator is responsible for the following tasks:

- creating the culture of the programme;
- representing the programme to the public and to the various collaborating agencies;

Figure 11.1
System model of
a national cancer
control programme

INPUTS ▶	PROCESSES ▶	OUTPUTS ▶	OUTCOMES
Resources	**How programme organizes resources**	**Direct products of programme activities**	**Impacts on the people participating in the programme**
• leadership • team • staff • partners • patients • written policies and plans • other programmes • money • facilities • supplies • organizations • knowledge • laws etc.	• the comprehensive programme is launched in a demonstration area • communication strategy, education and training are developed • a stepwise and systemic approach to implementing activities is used • existing resources are optimized, tailored to priority areas and needs for investments are assessed • training methodologies are applied to change established practices in the workplace and to improve effectiveness and efficiency of programme activities etc.	• number of people served by the programme • number of press conferences, documents targeting different audiences, progress reports, publications, etc. • steps accomplished, teams and interrelated processes in operation • amount of resources allocated, amount of new investments • number of health care workers trained and duration of training etc.	• modified attitudes, values and behaviours among the target population • increased knowledge, motivation and participation of customers, health professionals and other relevant stakeholders • increased motivation, new knowledge and skills, plus desired changes achieved among health care workers • improved survival rates • reduction in incidence and mortality rates • improved quality of life of patients and their families etc.

- providing assistance to the individuals responsible for the various programme activities;
- ensuring that activities and events are coordinated to gain maximum effect;
- ensuring that the programme is reviewed at regular intervals;
- setting targets for quality assurance and improvement.

The board of the national cancer control programme should amply represent all key sectors of the community. It should consist of the people responsible for various programme activities, whether governmental or nongovernmental, including oncology specialists and the general public. This multidisciplinary group should work as a team, led by the programme coordinator. The board should have a constitution that sets out its mandate, specifies its accountability, defines its membership, and specifies the frequency of its meetings.

The coordinator of the national cancer control programme should facilitate or reinforce the building of a network of local coordinators, backed by their own teams, who will take a leadership role in their areas or regions. Ideally, these local leaders should coordinate with the central organization, but keep their autonomy to administer their own resources and adjust national cancer control plans to their local situation.

The functions of the board of the national cancer control programme are given in Box 11.1.

Box 11.1 Functions of the board of a national cancer control programme

The board of a national cancer control programme should:

- oversee the development and revision of the written programme plan;
- assume responsibility for implementation of the plan;
- obtain political commitment from the government;
- coordinate the work of all agencies that can contribute to cancer control;
- oversee the systematic development and coordination of specific cancer control activities, such as prevention, early detection, treatment, and palliative care, so as to ensure the best use of available resources for the whole population;
- oversee financial aspects of the programme, including budgeting and fundraising;
- recommend legislative action to change cancer control policies;
- oversee public education and participation;
- oversee development of national diagnosis and treatment guidelines
- oversee professional education and development;
- identify and recommend research priorities;
- forecast future trends and coordinate the strategic development of health services, the health system, and the training and supply of health professionals;
- develop and support cancer control programmes for sub-populations within the country;
- recommend priorities for the investment of additional resources;
- develop a communication strategy;
- oversee the information systems;
- oversee the programme evaluation process, and implement corrective changes as needed.

Team building, or the ability to gather the right people and get them working together for the benefit of a project, is essential in a cancer control programme. Most of the managerial, clinical or community activities require teamwork. Effective teams are results-oriented and are committed to project objectives, milestones, goals and strategies. The team's behaviour is subject to socially acceptable standards that are shared by all members. In the work environment the most important standards relate to the group performance.

Characteristics of good team building include the following:

- team is clear about goals and established targets;
- each team member is willing to contribute;
- team leader has good interpersonal skills and is committed to team approach;
- high level of interdependence exists among team members;
- team develops a relaxed climate for communication;
- team members develop mutual trust;
- team and individuals are prepared to take risks;
- roles of team members are defined;
- team norms are defined;
- team members know how to examine team and individual errors without personal animosity;
- team has capacity to create new ideas;
- team members know that they can each influence the team agenda.

It is important to keep in mind the various barriers to team development. A high proportion of health professionals, who work mainly at the clinical level, may resist public health approaches. In addition, health managers and their team generally work in unfavourable conditions, have low salaries and have to perform competing tasks for other programmes. Motivating them and keeping them involved may constitute a major challenge. Meetings and training workshops should create an appropriate environment, so that the team—and especially new team members—understand the team's overall goal, their specific role within the team in contributing to the attainment of that goal, and the rationale for the public health strategies the team will be implementing. When resources are limited, there is a need to provide actively for psychosocial and cultural incentives, such as public and private acknowledgement of their efforts, enhancement of the contribution each team member plays in the achievement of the common goal, and continuous training.

The written plan for the national cancer control programme

Steps in development of the national cancer control programme were discussed in the previous chapter. Oversight of this process and the preparation of a written plan are the responsibility of the programme board, working by itself or through coordination of the work of various committees. The written plan should be formulated and tailored to the needs of the country. The following outline has served as a valuable model for national cancer control programme plans:

- assessment of the cancer situation;
- clear definition of goals and objectives
- identification of the priority needs of the country;
- outlining the strategies for cancer control;
- assessment of resources available and how they are organized in the health system;
- setting of achievable targets, and indicating by whom, when and where they are to be carried out.

Acceptance of the plan may be facilitated by drafting a discussion paper on cancer control, and circulating it for comment by the government and by nongovernmental organizations. Review and approval of a plan can be a lengthy process, but a draft plan that the board can use for lobbying may assist in speeding up the process. Copies of national cancer control programme plans and related materials for a number of developed and developing countries are available in the literature and on the Internet.

Written guidelines

For each priority area, evidence-based guidelines should be elaborated. These guidelines should be accepted by consensus, and must address clinical and management aspects, in order to standardize the procedures and contribute to quality assurance of the different activities.

Programmes that already exist

When the national cancer control plan and the priorities for initial cancer control activities have been agreed, the resources to implement the plan must be mobilized, either by bidding for new resources or by using existing resources. It may often be possible to mobilize existing resources that can be incorporated into the national cancer control programme or with which the programme can collaborate in order to maximize their usefulness. Linkages between existing cancer control activities and other programmes, such as those for the control of other non-communicable diseases, tobacco, sexually transmitted diseases/AIDS, nutrition, and environmental contamination, will be conducive to the primary prevention of cancer. Close coordination with hepatitis B virus vaccination programmes and schistosomiasis control projects should be planned in areas where these diseases present significant problems.

The national cancer control programme should be integrated into, and collaborate with, existing healthcare systems, both public and private, at the different levels of care, including hospitals, and primary health care clinics. The programme cannot, however, be run exclusively within any one of these levels, since activities will be concerned with different levels, or sometimes a combination of levels. Thus many primary prevention activities may be run largely within the primary healthcare level (for example, HBV immunization), whereas others, such as early detection and screening strategies, may involve all three levels. Diagnosis and treatment require a multidisciplinary approach, and coordination among the different disciplines should be enhanced to improve quality of care. Primary healthcare centres have a major role to play in public health education and early detection; medical, paramedical, and community care workers should be the resource persons for these activities, and an effective link in the referral chain. Active participation of primary health care workers is an important component of an effective cancer control programme.

Partnership

Partners who are engaged in the fight against cancer may come from governmental, nongovernmental, and private sectors, as well as professional organizations. All have the common objective of reducing cancer morbidity and mortality. Partners from each sector must play a role in the development of a national cancer control programme, though the relative extent of that role will vary from country to country. In close collaboration with WHO, the International Union Against Cancer (UICC) promotes the participation of nongovernmental organizations in the development and implementation of national (regional) cancer control plans, and helps to build capacity in the areas of cancer prevention and early detection, particularly through education and training programmes.

NGOs can often perform roles in cancer control that cannot be undertaken by government because of fiscal or political constraints. It is important to consult NGOs early in the development of a national cancer control programme in order to secure their collaboration. Particular areas of activity should be identified as the responsibility of government (for example, government is usually responsible for providing most health personnel and services), and others as the responsibility of NGOs. NGOs need to work within the national cancer control programme, and should avoid promoting measures that are appropriate in other countries but impractical in their own.

NGOs are involved in a variety of cancer control activities, ranging from research, registration, and prevention to treatment and patient care and facilities, either through direct provision of the services or as funding bodies. In some countries, funding for treatment comes from the central government, while funding for disease prevention and screening is provided by local government sources. In other countries, funding comes mostly from private sources, with NGOs playing a major role in initiating prevention and early detection activities. It is very important that all players are aware of the complexity of the national situation and of the role each can or should play to achieve the goals of a national cancer control programme. A comprehensive and systematic approach to the cancer problem, as presented in a national cancer control programme, gives all partners the opportunity of contributing their best to a unified endeavour.

The nongovernmental sector is an important source of technical know-how, expertise, and resources, and provides outreach to the professional and public communities. The need for community participation in cancer control and patient care is evident. This need is particularly acute in developing countries, given the resource constraints and operational limitations of their governmental health care systems. In many countries, major portions of their healthcare budgets are dedicated to the control of communicable diseases, leaving little for allocation to noncommunicable diseases. Nongovernmental and voluntary organizations should, therefore, play a significant role in reducing disparities in the level of cancer prevention, early detection and patient care that governmental health systems are able to provide.

A budget for cancer control

In drawing up the budget of the national cancer control programme, it is useful to start by identifying all the budgets currently used for every aspect of cancer control. Bodies already active in related activities may be defensive about their budgets, but should understand that there may be opportunities for the reallocation or sharing of resources in the future, when the national programme has developed a sense of common purpose. Even if precise budgetary information is not available, it is useful to estimate current expenditure on each of the four major strategy components: primary prevention, early diagnosis and screening, treatment (surgery, radiotherapy and chemotherapy), and palliative care. Based upon agreement within the national cancer control programme board on priorities, and with the relevant agencies, resources should be reallocated from unproductive areas to areas with greater potential for success.

In general, resources for the national cancer control programme should be provided by the government and supplemented by NGOs and, if necessary, by special fundraising. Since the establishment of a national cancer control programme is intended to increase the priority given to cancer control in the country's health care programme; to raise the profile of those working in cancer control; and to increase the resources devoted to cancer control; it is probable that the availability of funds within the country concerned will increase. The very process of developing a national cancer control programme will facilitate the mobilization of funds and may increase the accessibility of funds within the country. In addition, international donors are likely to be attracted by a well-conceived programme that promises to increase the efficiency and effectiveness of cancer control. Fund-raising from these and other sources is a major part of the responsibilities of the programme coordinator and board.

Information systems

Information systems should be developed in order to monitor the programme processes and indicate ad hoc changes to improve them. For example, effective patient care requires timely diagnosis, treatment and adequate follow-up. A good information system should be able to identify delays or bottlenecks in the system, and impediments to follow-up and adherence so that such problems can be readily solved. Ideal, comprehensive, information systems can be very costly and difficult to maintain. In limited resource settings, information systems should be tailored to the basic needs of the selected priorities, and carefully developed to ensure the monitoring and evaluation of key process components and outcome measures in the priority areas. Information systems should be linked to population-based cancer registries in the areas where they exist so outcome measures such as incidence, stage distribution and survival can be provided by the surveillance system. Sample survey methods can be used to supplement this approach.

Legislation

In some countries, legislation may be needed to provide the necessary authority for those who are to run the national cancer control programme. In others, legislation may have to be introduced or amended to allow the costs of some activities (for example, screening tests) to be covered by the government or by health insurance schemes.

Which are key processes for a national cancer control programme to fulfil its goals?

Processes should be managed to meet the requirements and needs of customers, providers and other stakeholders. Clear roles and responsibilities must be established for managing the process and the interrelations with functions of other processes or programmes must be identified as well. The processes must align with the national cancer control programme objectives and should include continual improvement of performance. Decisions and actions should be based on the analysis of data and information to improve results, and not rely merely on opinions as usually occurs.

The following paragraphs describe some key processes that are useful to consider when implementing or reorienting a national cancer control programme. These processes are based on principles of quality management as well as on practical experiences at the country level.

Launching the programme

A successful launch can facilitate public acceptance of a national cancer control programme, increase the understanding of the principles underlying the programme, and rally support for its strategies. Once the programme plan has been developed, consideration can be given to the approaches to be used for launching the programme. If only minimal resistance is anticipated and if there is confidence that the planned strategies can be successfully implemented nationally, the programme board can move directly to a launch with a national conference. This implies careful planning and involvement of media experts. From the beginning, the board needs to work closely with the media experts and others preparing all aspects of the conference, including press releases, brochures, and other background material, and ensuring that such material is acceptable to the government and the NGOs involved. If any resistance is anticipated, careful analysis of the situation is needed to identify the barriers and the possible mechanisms for overcoming them. In some cases it is preferable to focus the programme initially in a demonstration area.

Demonstration areas

Experience gained by various countries show that it is often advisable to start small and consider that success breeds success. Efforts can concentrate on a demonstration area, which has a good likelihood of successfully implementing one or two priority initiatives that can serve as entry points. Thus political and financial support can be enhanced and the expansion of the programme both geographically and thematic can be considered in a second stage, once concrete achievements can be demonstrated.

Sustained communication strategy

The board of the national cancer control programme should oversee the development of a sustained communication strategy to support the implementation and progress of the programme, bearing in mind the following questions:

- whom do we wish to inform or influence;
- how often to communicate;
- by what means to communicate most cost-effectively;
- whether to publish a newsletter;
- whether to publish reports on cancer control;
- how to use an annual report to best effect.

Step-by-step implementation

A step-by-step process is recommended when starting or reorienting a cancer control programme, especially in a developing country setting. Implementation of a cancer control programme may proceed in a series of stages, each stage having clear measurable objectives and representing the basis for the development of the next stage, thereby permitting visible and controlled progress. Every stage should involve decision-makers and operational staff from the different levels of care that need to participate actively.

Optimizing existing resources from the start

Quite often, priority setting is neglected or does not follow the proper methodology. Scarce resources may not be well allocated or distributed. They may not be targeted to the right population group and they may be misused. There may be a lack of training and quality control. Thus, it is essential that at the first stage the programme considers reallocation of existing resources according to the new strategies, and foresees the development and incorporation of new technologies that are cost-effective, sustainable and of benefit to the majority of the targeted population.

Organizing activities of the priority areas with a systemic approach

Activities carried out according to the selected priorities should be tailored to the populations at risk. The activities should be adequately organized so as to make the best use of the available resources. Furthermore, it is important to take a systemic approach to ensure that the various interrelated components of the intervention strategy that share common objectives, are coordinated, directed to achieving the objectives, and integrated with other related programme or initiatives. An example of such an organization approach for a cervical cancer screening programme was given in Figure 10.3. Different components at various levels of care are essential and complementary parts of the system. All these components need to be managed efficiently in order to guarantee quality and their permanent coordination. They also need to be continuously monitored to achieve reduction in incidence and mortality from invasive cancer. Furthermore, each component is a subsystem with its own particular management process. At the primary level of care, where the majority of the women at risk are screened, the activities are integrated with programmes of reproductive health, other preventive clinical services and community-outreach initiatives. At the secondary and tertiary levels the components are integrated with the hospital services that provide diagnosis, treatment, and eventually, palliative care to the cases that were not detected early by the system.

Education and training

Ideally, health professionals, including nurses, doctors and health managers, should have some public health training during their undergraduate and post-graduate courses. Such training should give healthcare providers knowledge and skills in epidemiology, screening, and health services organization and management. Programmes to educate and train health care professionals, consumers, and other stakeholders should be tailored to the type of audience, the local situation and the momentum in the national cancer control programme development so as to ensure that they contribute to improving the programme. The teaching of behavioural modification skills should be encouraged, as many aspects of cancer prevention, treatment and palliative care require behavioural changes from the public, the patient and the health worker.

One way of establishing a broad base of support and improving programme performance, is to hold a national problem-solving workshop with the participation of professionals from all related disciplines and from all levels of the health system, covering all the targeted administrative areas. The goal of the workshop could be to strengthen national capacity to manage cancer control programmes. The initiative includes follow-up meetings to reinforce the processes generated by the initial workshop.

Continuous training of health care workers needs to be developed along the lines of quality management. That is, it should focus on active involvement, continual improvement and innovation and creativity. Such training is key to achieving the desired changes in behaviour in line with new policies, and thus to improve the performance of the programme.

Spiral of problem solving and team learning methodology

This is an example of a learning methodology that can be used to improve the effectiveness and efficiency of a public health programme by changing established practices in the workplace. A common problem encountered in the implementation of a national cancer control programme is how to produce a change in the established practices of professional workers. The spiral of problem solving and team learning is an effective methodology to deal with this situation (Salas 2001). This methodology is a combination of problem-based learning methodology (Barrows and Tamblyn 1980) and the study of work for better decision-making (Sketchley et al. 1986). The approach is designed to give ownership of the process to the local manager and team by promoting their active participation in planning, implementation, monitoring and evaluation. The basic assumptions underlying this approach are that:

- health workers can learn from their workplace experiences;
- human and material resources already in use can be redirected through low cost intervention to produce a more efficient programme;
- formal lines of authority in the public health sector must be respected to minimize resistance and improve potential support;
- existing levels of authority are interested in improving the programme when they are involved, respected, motivated, trained and supported.

The methodological principles governing this intervention concern both personal and collective components. The first personal principle is that programme leaders must begin by changing themselves before asking others around them to change. Individuals perceive obstacles as limiting their possible choices, so an important principle is to stop that restrictive attitude and think of obstacles as an opportunity for creativity. Another important personal principle is to learn not only from personal experience, but from everyone, thus people should always be open to new ideas. Further, each person deserves respect and appreciation, so rejection and criticism should be avoided.

As a collective, the group always needs to keep the big picture in mind, continuously aware of what part is taking place at any given time. The objective should always be clarified first, and then the plan of action should be designed to achieve that objective. Another important principle is that the use of available resources should be optimized first, before consideration of adding any new resources. Similarly, the focus of the group should be teamwork, using the skills and talents of existing staff. When an outline of any plan is developed, part of the plan should always be left open to allow the local team to make adjustments and to innovate. Lastly, the process needs to be sustained with high quality information, with the teams taking an active part in collecting, interpreting and disseminating the information.

A cycle of the spiral of problem solving and team learning methodology has an internal phase and a public or external phase. During the internal phase an expert team plans a project. During the public phase, the participants work at the managerial and operation levels to implement and evaluate the project. Initially, the expert team identifies the problems and drafts a general sequence for solving them. Then it selects one specific problem and develops a plan. The plan should have a fixed framework, providing opportunities for input from the health managers and teams. Subsequently, a public phase is initiated, consisting of the following steps:

- invitation of the established responsible managers to a short workshop, usually one day; this respects the existing hierarchy and develops a critical mass that will positively influence others.
- the initial short workshop should be carefully designed and implemented so as to create the momentum to initiate the programme and obtain the commitment of the participants. The workshop includes a presentation from an expert clearly identifying the problem; the managers and their teams work to analyse the shortcomings and suggest solutions, following written guidelines; the teams are taught the essential skills for solving the problem, generally through demonstrations; the teams are given guidance on how to present the results of the field work; and the teams are invited to develop solutions to the problem in their own workplace and present the results at the next workshop.
- the teams return to their place of work, pursue their plan of action in their health establishment using local creativity to solve the problem, and collect information on the results;
- at the next short workshop, teams make oral presentations of their results; successes and innovation are recognized; and as soon as the presentations are finished, the same workshop starts the next cycle of problem-solving, building on the successful solution of the previous problem.

The strategy is described schematically in Figure 11.2.

Consequently, the staff is involved in "learning by doing". This is done in a gradual way or successive cycles, going from the simplest to the most complex, from the inner environment (healthcare services) to the outside environment (community outreach). Initially, the cycle

Figure 11.2
Spiral of problem-solving and team learning at the workplace

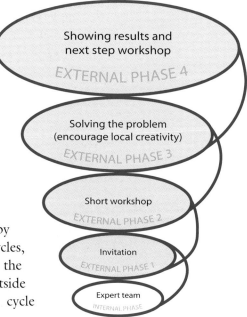

Showing results and next step workshop
EXTERNAL PHASE 4

Solving the problem (encourage local creativity)
EXTERNAL PHASE 3

Short workshop
EXTERNAL PHASE 2

Invitation
EXTERNAL PHASE 1

Expert team
INTERNAL PHASE

143

typically focuses on the health service officials themselves. For example, if the problem were related to reducing smoking rates, the initial cycle would involve reducing the smoking rate of health care professionals and promoting non-smoking in indoor premises. Likewise, if the problem were related to cervical cancer screening, the initial cycle would be the screening of female personnel of the health care centres. Then the cycles are expanded step-wise to eventually reach the general public. In the example of cervical cancer screening (see Figure 11.3), the expanding set of cycles include the quality control of the Pap smear samples, which is addressed using the same approach.

The reorganization of the cervical cytology screening programme in Chile, a middle-income country, is given as an example of this methodology (Box 11.2). In this example, each cycle was accomplished in 3 to 8 months. In the first cycle, from July to October 1988, the Pap smear coverage of women, aged 25–64, working at the primary health centres of the Metropolitan Region of Santiago, increased from 41% to 79%.

Constraints in moving from policy to implementation

The challenge for the national cancer control programme is to provide guidance compatible with the scientific evidence, in order to justify cancer control endeavours within the context of fiscal and other constraints. Implementation of a national cancer control programme means facing up to issues such as health sector reform, health care financing, globalization, and the impact of various financial policies that are forcing cuts in social service spending. Further, given the scarcity of resources, the focus on high priority public health problems, in particular HIV/AIDS, must be taken into account.

In some countries, especially in the least developed ones, implementation will be slow. Sometimes cancer

Figure 11.3
Expanding cycles—
cervical cancer

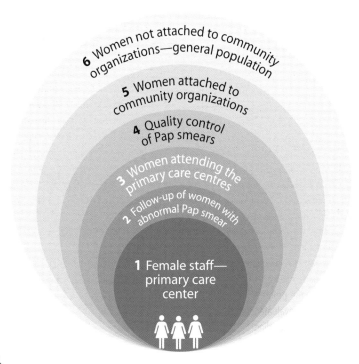

6 Women not attached to community organizations—general population
5 Women attached to community organizations
4 Quality control of Pap smears
3 Women attending the primary care centres
2 Follow-up of women with abnormal Pap smear
1 Female staff—primary care center

control activities will take place outside the concept of a national cancer control programme. In other countries comprehensive tobacco control interventions may move ahead independently because of political will, and because their justification is wider than cancer, involving cardiovascular and respiratory diseases and maternal and child health as well. In some countries, the implementation of a national cervical screening programme may be linked to maternal, child and women's health, although in such a case, it may be difficult to ensure that priorities reside with the screening of women over the age of 35 years.

Frequently, health initiatives do not address the thorny question of collaboration. It is left to front line primary care providers to work out how to collaborate when they are confronted with multiple guidelines and protocols on how to deal with the management of childhood illnesses, safe

---

Box 11.2 Reorganization of the cervical cancer screening programme in Chile

In 1985, with the assistance of WHO, a national cancer control programme was founded at the Ministry of Health, with cervical cancer as one of the main priorities.

Over the two previous decades, opportunistic annual screening for cervical cancer had not achieved the expected reduction in mortality. Therefore, in 1987, a public health oriented cervical screening programme was launched, based on screening women aged 25 to 64 with a Pap smear every three years. Unfortunately many health professionals were reluctant to apply the ministry's approach. Consequently, efforts and resources were initially focused on the Santiago Metropolitan Region, which constitutes one third of the population, as a demonstration area. Seven years later, the programme was expanded to the remainder of the country.

The programme emphasized network organization; timeliness of diagnosis and treatment (more than 80% of women with abnormal Pap smears get prompt medical attention); reliability of Pap smear (100% of public laboratories are included in an external quality control system), and low cost screening promotion strategies at the community level. An information system covering the women

entering the programme was implemented and included case registries in every level of the health system.

During the initial years, the financial support for the programme was minimal. Additional funding from the government was provided after 6 years to upgrade equipment at the secondary level, and to support community-based, low cost promotion activities.

The strategy adopted in the Metropolitan Area, which was later applied to the rest of the country, included involvement of health authorities and a series of training workshops for health professionals concerned with the programme at each level of care. The workshops were conducted with the help of a physician who was an expert in education and health communication. In each workshop, the participants received motivational input and updated information on the programme. They were trained how to assess the current situation, how to compare it to the desired one, and how to develop specific strategies to bridge the existing gaps. After a few months, in the next workshop, the progress and constraints encountered were evaluated and subsequent tasks were planned accordingly.

The first strategy implemented was motivation of female health care providers within the health care system to be screened.

The second strategy was monitoring the follow-up of women with abnormal Pap smears in the different levels of care. Different process indicators were evaluated, such as compliance and timeliness of diagnosis and treatment, quality control of cytology, information system, and coordination among different programme components. Serious weaknesses were encountered, and for several months all efforts focused on reorganization before invitations to women to be screened were issued widely.

The third and fourth strategies offered screening to women in the target group. Promotion to invite women attending primary health care centres for screening was followed by community strategies to reach older women. These activities were carefully synchronized with health centres to ensure adequate provision of care.

Coverage of the target group by Pap smear rose from 40% in 1990 to 66% in 1997. The age-adjusted mortality rate for cancer of the cervix decreased from 13.3 per 100 000 women in 1970 to 7.7 per 100 000 women in 1999.

motherhood, HIV/AIDS, tuberculosis, cancer, reproductive health, and so on. If specialists with years of training cannot integrate their work, it will be difficult for a primary health care provider; often under-trained and usually under-supported, to do so.

Countries with unstable economies and politics often face competing priorities for social and health actions, thus affecting their ability to plan and implement national programmes. In addition, their often-insufficient financial, technical, and human resources deleteriously affect national interventions. In many countries, there is limited organizational and management capacity for cancer control within Ministries of Health. Furthermore, evidence on cost-effective preventive, early detection and treatment methods may not be accessible to national health authorities. Without basic tools for assessment, such as surveillance systems and cancer registries, many countries will not have the capacity for accurate monitoring and evaluation of interventions.

Many of these constraints to planning and implementing a national cancer control programme can be counteracted by good management that ensures the selection of adequate priorities. Effective management will also ensure that the right methodologies are applied in the right place at the right time with the right people and within the framework of a national cancer control programme. Good management will focus on: goal orientation; the needs of customers; effective leadership and partnership; active involvement of all stakeholders; the promotion of political will; rational planning, innovative and creative approaches; effective and efficient stepwise implementation; continuous training; problem solving and behavioural change; monitoring progress and outcomes; and a systemic, comprehensive approach. International cooperation and global initiatives, also play a major role in supporting initiatives at country level.

GLOBAL ACTION TO SUPPORT NATIONAL EFFORTS

WHO and other United Nations technical and development agencies can assist countries with national cancer control programme infrastructure development, strategy development, management issues, manpower training and research capacity building. A number of programmes and activities have been developed for broader health purposes, and these provide a context in which cancer control activities can, and should, be developed. Resources can be used most efficiently if activities are well coordinated to avoid duplication of effort. This is especially important in developing countries, where funds are particularly limited. Global actions, focusing on the reduction of risk, the improvement of treatment, and the training of health professionals are described below and can provide support for the development of effective national cancer control programmes.

Alliances for healthy lifestyles, healthy environments and cancer control

WHO is promoting an integrated approach for the prevention and control of noncommunicable diseases. In Europe, the WHO CINDI programme (Countrywide Integrated Noncommunicable Diseases Intervention programme) advocates coordinated, comprehensive action to target common risk factors and unhealthy lifestyles, such as tobacco and alcohol use, physical inactivity, and obesity. In Latin America, the CARMEN programme (Conjunte de Acciones para Reduccion Multifactorial de Enfermedades No Transmissibles) promotes the adaptation of the same strategies and aims. Through a WHO Global Forum on Noncommunicable Diseases, WHO and its partners are working to establish similar networks for integrated noncommunicable diseases prevention in the other WHO regions: Africa, Eastern Mediterranean, South East Asia and the Western Pacific.

In the area of food safety WHO provides assessments of carcinogenic chemicals present in food through joint expert committees with the Food and Agriculture Organization of the United Nations (FAO). The results are used by the Codex Alimenatrius Commission to establish international food standards. In the field of environmental health risks, a comprehensive risk assessment of carcinogenic chemicals is undertaken by the International Programme on Chemical Safety (IPCS) and the joint programme of WHO, the International Labour Organization (ILO) and the United Nations Environment Programme (UNEP).

In order to promote a healthy diet on the basis of the most up-to-date scientific evidence, joint WHO/FAO expert consultations elaborate guidelines on diet, nutrition and the prevention of chronic diseases including cancer.

Intersun, WHO's global UV project, in cooperation with the United Nations Environment Programme, the World Meteorological Organization, the International Agency on Cancer Research and the International Commission on Non-Ionizing Radiation, aims to reduce the global burden of disease, including skin cancer, resulting from exposure to ultraviolet radiation. The programme encourages and evaluates research to fill gaps in scientific knowledge, assesses and quantifies health risks, and facilitates public and occupational programmes to reduce UV radiation-related health risks.

Framework convention for tobacco control

In 1999, based on a resolution adopted unanimously by the World Health Assembly, WHO took a leadership role in strengthening global tobacco control. It did this by initiating a process of multilateral negotiations between WHO Member States on a set of rules and regulations aimed towards governing the global rise and spread of tobacco. The Framework Convention on Tobacco Control (FCTC) will be an international legal instrument to improve transnational tobacco control. Once the Convention is adopted and enters into force, State Parties will take appropriate measures to fulfil the objectives and guiding principles of the convention through provisions which could address advertising and promotion, product regulation, elimination of illicit trade, and protection from exposure to environmental tobacco smoke, among others. Since the pre-negotiation phase concluded in 2000, four sessions of the Intergovernmental Negotiating Body have been held and significant progress has been achieved. The target date for adoption of the FCTC by the World Health Assembly is May 2003. The process is on schedule and Member States have reiterated the need to meet the deadline for the adoption of the Convention.

Immunization

For many years, infant vaccination has been recognized as a cost-effective approach to preventing life-threatening infections. Extension of these vaccination programmes to include the major oncogenic types of infectious agents associated with cancer could have a large impact on the global cancer burden, particularly if made available to populations where other prevention strategies are unavailable or not affordable. Liver cancer, the fifth most common cancer worldwide in males, has been shown to be associated with chronic infection with hepatitis B virus. The efficacy of hepatitis B vaccines against chronic infection exceeds 85% in regions where child and adult infection predominate. Hepatitis B vaccine is included in routine infant vaccination programmes in 135 of the 241 countries that report to WHO. International support and extension of WHO efforts to promote infant vaccination would not only be beneficial regarding the life-threatening infections to which they are directly targeted, but would also reduce the incidence of one of the most common cancers.

International efforts are being undertaken to support the development of new vaccines to help control other infections and their associated cancers. Of particular interest are the human papillomavirus (HPV) vaccines to control cervical cancer and *Helicobacter pylori* vaccines to reduce stomach cancer, both among the most common cancers worldwide.

Drug availability

WHO has identified essential drugs for cancer treatment and palliative care. The 17 essential drugs for treatment are those that alone, or in conjunction with other therapeutic measures, will result in cure for some patients or a prolongation of survival for others. A WHO survey of 167 countries indicated that anti-neoplastic drugs were only available in 60% and affordable in less than half of those countries. In order to make these essential drugs available and affordable, national authorities need to develop national plans of action. WHO and other organizations can assist by identifying mechanisms to improve access, reduce costs and, where feasible, promote the local production of the essential agents.

Most of the strong painkillers are opioid analgesics that are subject to international control as narcotic drugs. Previous studies indicate that overly stringent regulations can reduce the availability of controlled drugs for medical use, such as oral morphine, a key to providing relief from cancer pain. To improve access to opioid analgesics, WHO is promoting balanced regulatory approaches so that control measures do not unduly restrict access to opioids. WHO has developed guidelines to assist national authorities to conduct self-diagnoses of their regulatory systems and identify any deficiencies that might exist. WHO also promotes a balanced opioids control policy through national and international workshops. In this regard, WHO is working with the International Narcotics Control Board, which has endorsed the above mentioned guidelines.

Strengthening cancer treatment facilities in least developed countries

Only about 50% of the population of Africa has access to radiation oncology services (Levin, 1999). The African Regional Agreement (AFRA) supported by the International Atomic Energy Agency (IAEA) is promoting the improvement of clinical radiotherapy in Africa by identifying areas with greatest need, facilitating equipment provision and sponsoring training. External assistance in this and other regions is needed to speed the pace of provision of these basic services. Of particular importance is the donation of diagnostic imaging and teletherapy equipment. Success in this area, however, depends on the informed commitment of the recipient countries and a commitment to long-term support, both for equipment and infrastructure, on the part of the donor.

Human resources for cancer control

Most developing countries lack an adequate number of professionals to staff their cancer control services according to the results of the WHO assessment of the national capacity for non communicable disease prevention and control (WHO, 2001b). Often, both an increase in the number of specialists and improved training are needed. Areas of professional specialization in cancer control include not only diagnosis and treatment, but also disease prevention, early detection, palliative care, and research. For many years WHO, IARC and other international organizations have been actively involved in the development of human resources for cancer control. The number of individuals trained in these initiatives is, however, still woefully short of what is needed. Additional organizations need to join this effort in order to ensure that basic training needs are met, while avoiding excessive specialization and sophistication.

Even in industrialized countries, human resources for cancer control need to be improved. Although tobacco is the most preventable cause of ill-health in the world today, few schools of public health offer specialization or even courses in tobacco control.

Promotion of reliable information

The quality of medical care depends on the quality and availability of information. A number of sources, including prestigious institutions and the major medical journals, provide reliable, peer-reviewed information. A great deal of information is available regarding basic, epidemiological and clinical research, but far less is available in the applied public health field, especially from a developing country perspective. International efforts are being undertaken to promote quality standards for reliable information on the World Wide Web. There are also initiatives aimed at providing greater access to reliable information, especially for professionals in developing countries, by making peer-reviewed journals available free or at reduced cost. WHO has brokered an agreement among the world's leading publishers of medical journals to provide online access to their journals free or almost free to developing countries. In order to promote the technical preconditions needed to access information online, WHO is spearheading the United Nation Health InterNetwork project.

MONITORING AND EVALUATING THE PROGRAMME

12

WHAT IS PROGRAMME EVALUATION?

Programme evaluation is "the systematic assessment of the operation and/or outcomes of a programme or policy compared to a set of explicit or implicit standards, as a means of contributing to the improvement of the programme or policy" (Weiss, 1998). Continuous evaluation of processes and outcomes of a national cancer control programme is an essential tool for assessing its organizational progress and enhancing its effectiveness. Evaluation is also necessary for fulfilling its operational principles as described in Chapter 10.

HOW TO CARRY OUT EFFECTIVE EVALUATION OF A NATIONAL CANCER CONTROL PROGRAMME?

Any programme evaluation requires careful design and planning that should start early in the process of programming. There is abundant literature on evaluation regarding design, combination of methods and techniques of analysis. A comprehensive framework for programme evaluation (Centers for Disease Control, 1999) is adapted here to guide the process of evaluating a national cancer control programme. The following key questions should be formulated when planning an evaluation and later on when reviewing its implementation:

- Who will evaluate?
- What will be evaluated?
- How should the evaluation be designed and implemented?
- By what means can the credibility of the evidence gathered be enhanced?
- What standards (type or level of performance) must be reached for the national cancer control programme to be considered successful?
- What conclusions regarding the national cancer control programme performance are justified by comparing available evidence to the standards?
- How will lessons learnt from the results of the evaluation be used to improve the national cancer control programme performance?

Who will evaluate?

The national cancer control programme coordinator and the board should take the lead in planning and implementing the evaluation and should ensure that the relevant stakeholders are involved throughout the whole process. These include those involved in the programmes's operations, those served by the national cancer control programme, and primary users of the evaluation. If stakeholders are not involved, the evaluation might overlook key elements of the programme and thus its findings might be ignored or resisted. Involving stakeholders should consider their perspectives, skills and concerns. Different expertise or complementary competencies can enrich the process and make the evaluation more effective. For example, social and behavioural scientists can be instrumental in helping to analyse how the programme operates in the organizational and community contexts. Creative thinking can help ensure the results of the evaluation influence the decision-making process in the right direction.

What will be evaluated?

The programme coordinator, the board and relevant stakeholders should decide what will be systematically evaluated in the national cancer control programme. It should include the national cancer control programme and its context. A thorough description of the programme will ensure that there is an understanding of programme goals, strategies, resources, stages of development, sociopolitical context and the programme's capacity to produce change. It is useful to construct a logic model that synthesizes the main programme elements and gives a picture of how the programme is supposed to work. Such a model improves and focuses programme direction. Examples of such models were given in Figures 10.3 and 11.2 in the previous chapters.

How should the evaluation be designed and implemented?

The evaluation design depends on the purposes of the evaluation, the users, and the resources available to carry out the evaluation. The more an evaluation is focused on the concerns of stakeholders the more efficient it will be in ensuring that the findings of the evaluation will be used as intended. Consideration of the questions to be answered and the units of analysis are essential in selecting methods and gathering evidence.

Evaluation activities are part of a continuum of actions that support the decision-making process in all stages of programming: planning, implementation and outcome evaluation. Evaluation is thus useful to all programme activities and provides a wide scope for evidence-based decisions within a national cancer control programme (Brazil, 1999).

Programme monitoring

Monitoring is intended to assess whether the implementation of a national cancer control programme is performing as was devised, and whether or not the programme is reaching the target population and meeting the needs of customers.

Suitable criteria for overall evaluation of a national cancer control programme in its early stages are:

- the endorsement by the Ministry of Health and key NGOs of the concept of a national cancer control programme, with a commitment to provide the necessary political and financial support;
- the existence of a defined budget to enable the programme to support initiatives;
- the existence of a clear plan and measures that can be used to judge progress in implementation of the plan;
- the appointment of a programme coordinator and board and the allocation of sufficient resources to support the work;
- a written programme of work that assigns clear roles and responsibilities, and covers the following issues:
  - prevention;
  - early diagnosis and treatment;
  - palliative care;
  - monitoring and evaluation systems.

Once a national cancer control programme is more advanced in its implementation or is well established, programme performance can be assessed by different methods, depending on how comprehensive an evaluation is required (organization, prevention, early detection, treatment and palliative care) and on which quality dimensions are included for controlling the processes. Performance measurements are useful tools for continual quality improvement initiatives. They are used to establish the baseline level of performance and to re-measure the performance level after quality improvement has been done.

The classical approach to the assessment of quality is through structure, process and outcome measures (Donabedian 1980). *Structure measures* evaluate resources available in the programme; *Process measures* evaluate the workings of, and interactions between, the various components of a programme; *Outcome measures* evaluate the effects of a programme on the population that are expected to have short, medium or long-term consequences, depending on the nature of the processes involved. Examples of structure, process and outcome measures are summarized in Table 12.1.

These measures can be evaluated in the system model of inputs, processes, outputs and outcomes—elements that were analysed in Chapter 11. It is important that evaluation of a national cancer control programme encompasses leadership, stakeholder's involvement, and partnerships; as well as how policies, plans, products and services are managed, updated and delivered. The above methodology facilitates scrutiny of all those issues. Monitoring and setting appropriate information systems, such as that discussed for cervical screening (Miller 1992), is very important in ensuring that implementation will produce efficient and timely outputs. Tracking systems will be required for prevention and for service delivery in relation to screening, treatment and palliative care. Continuous monitoring and analysis of operational and financial data – which can be facilitated by the use of appropriate computer programs – not only highlight the areas of the national cancer control programme that should be modified, but

Table 12.1 Evaluation of a national cancer control programme

Evaluation category	Programme	Primary prevention	Early detection and screening	Treatment	Palliative care
Structure measures	Published plan endorsed by ministry of health	Agency or consortium identified responsible for health promotion	Policy agreed upon for education for early detection	Guidelines on treatment agreed	Pain relief policy adopted
	Programme coordinator and board appointed	Sampling surveys of risk factor prevalence performed	Organized screening programmes planned for priority cancers	Essential drug list for chemotherapy adopted	Education of health professionals Legislation passed to ensure availability of oral morphine
Process measures	Collaboration obtained for programmes with relevant government ministries and NGOs	Anti-tobacco education in >80% of schools >70% of infants HBV vaccinated	>80% of people aware of warning signs for cancer >80% of people in target groups examined once	>70% of patients treated according to guidelines >20% of cancer patients receive curative treatment	Trends in morphine and other opioids consumption >50% of general hospitals adopt WHO guidelines
Short-term outcomes (within 5 years)	Substantially increased knowledge of cancer obtained in all relevant sectors	Significant reduction in exposure to risk factors in the general population	>30% of cancers detected on examination or by tests	>50% of cancer patients survive one year	>40% of cancer patients in pain are relieved from pain
Medium-term outcomes (within 10 years)	Effect of programme shown on cancer incidence	Reduction in incidence of other diseases (e.g. cardiovascular, respiratory)	>30% reduction in targeted advanced cancers	>30% of cancer patients survive 5 years	Quality of life is improved in >60% of patients
Long-term outcomes (15–20 years)	>15% of reduction in peak cancer mortality	Reduction in incidence of relevant cancers (e.g. lung) has begun	>15% reduction in mortality for targeted cancers	>10% reduction in cancer mortality attributable to treatment	Quality of life is improved in >80% of patients

also provide the information feedback required by government ministries and other funding agencies. For instance, data on the costs per patient of an intervention at a particular stage of a particular cancer can be linked to future projections of patient loads, or to data on the number and type of inpatient and outpatient visits and treatments. This would provide a wealth of information for programme budgeting and for estimation of the equipment, personnel, and accommodation needed by treatment facilities.

In the context of continuous quality improvement (CQI), which focuses mainly on the needs of customers, team work and continual improvement of performance, quality is described and measured according to a number of dimensions including accessibility, appropriateness, efficiency and effectiveness (Canadian Council On Health Services Accreditation, 1996). This type of evaluation impacts everyone, from senior management to operational staff. Examples of quality dimension and their possible performance indicators for prevention, early detection, treatment and palliation are illustrated in Table 12.2.

Outcome evaluation

Once a national cancer control programme becomes established and has a regular budget, it is important to assess its overall effectiveness. Outcome indicators comprise the impacts on the people receiving the services of the programme. For a national cancer control programme, these indicators are concerned with the quality of life of cancer patients, disease recurrence rates, disease-free survival rates, overall survival rates among treated patients, incidence, and mortality rates. Reliable baseline data on the common types of cancer, their stage at diagnosis, and the outcome of disease are essential if valid programme outcome measures are to be set. It is therefore important that data collection systems are developed as early in the programme as possible. Where they exist, population-based cancer registries will yield valuable material for this purpose and can provide a continuous input of epidemiological data.

The best way of assessing programme outcomes is by means of a randomized experimental design, which compares the results of the programme to a control group. However, most outcome evaluations cannot use this model, and have to rely on quasi-experimental designs to ensure that the outcomes can be attributed to the programme. Assessment of programme efficiency, on the other hand, relies on analysis of cost–benefit, cost–effectiveness, and cost–utility. An efficient programme is one that achieves the best possible results using the available resources. A programme that seems likely to have a significant impact on a country's cancer problems is of little value if the resources required to sustain it exceed those that can be made available.

Table 12.2: Examples of quality dimensions that can be used to evaluate the performance of a national cancer control programme

Quality Dimensions in the performance of a national cancer control programme	Example of indicators for smoking cessation programme	Example of indicators for cervical cancer screening (including treatment)	Example of indicators for treatment of curable cancers	Example of indicators for palliative care
Acceptability *How well the health system is meeting expectations of the providers and the public*	• Level of satisfaction of providers and patients with tobacco cessation counselling in the workplace	• Level of satisfaction of providers and patients with the screening programme	• Level of satisfaction of providers and patients with the treatment	• Level of satisfaction of providers and patients with the palliative care programme
Accessibility *Whether or not the public and patients can obtain the preventive and control services they need at the right place and time*	• Percentage of providers and patients who are smokers that have access to tobacco cessation counselling	• Percentage of at risk women with a Pap smear taken in the last 5 years • Timeliness of diagnosis and treatment for patients referred for having an abnormal cytology	• Percentage of patients with curable cancers that receive adequate treatment • Timeliness of diagnosis and treatment of cases referred for having warning signs	• Level of morphine and other opioids consumption • Percentage of cancer patients with advanced cancer who have access to palliative care services
Appropriateness *Whether care is relevant to the needs and is based on established standards*	• Percentage of patients with a non-communicable disease that are assessed about their tobacco smoking status	• Quality of Pap smears taken by primary health care workers and gynaecologists • Percentage of patients with pre-cancerous cervical lesions that are treated with non-invasive procedures	• Percentage of patients that are treated according to guidelines	• Percentage of patients who receive palliative care according to guidelines
Competence *Whether the knowledge and skills of providers are appropriate to the services that they are providing*	• Percentage of primary health care workers with the necessary skills to give counselling on smoking cessation	• Continuing training of primary health care workers and laboratory staff regarding Pap smears collection, processing and analysis	• Quality assurance activities for diagnosis and treatment of the most common cancers	• Percentage of primary healthcare workers with the skills to provide basic palliative care
Continuity *How services fit together—coordination, integration, and ease of navigation*	• Plans implemented for avoiding relapse in ex-tobacco smokers	• Plans for follow-up of target population to repeat screening every 5 years • Follow-up mechanisms for patients treated for non-invasive cancer	• Mechanisms for long-term follow-up of treated patients	• Percentage of patients that have access to a trained health care worker in palliative care in their community
Effectiveness *How well services work and how they affect health status of the population at risk of cancer or affected by cancer*	• Tobacco cessation rates among smokers with low to severe addiction	• Changes in stage distribution of cervical cancer • Incidence of invasive cancer • Mortality from cervical cancer	• Overall and stage-specific survival rates	• Improved control of symptoms in patients with advanced cancer • Improved quality of life
Efficiency *Achieving best results at lowest cost*	• Costs of counselling	• Percentage of Pap smears taken from at risk women	• Comparative data on cost of treatments • Reduction in hospital stays	• Reduction of invasive procedures • Reduction in hospital stays
Safety *Minimizing potential risks of a health environment or service*	• Regulations to avoid passive smoking in healthcare settings	• Regulations to protect laboratory staff	• Radiation protection for patients and providers in radiotherapy services	• Measures to avoid abuse of opioids

By what means can the credibility of the evidence gathered be enhanced?

The following are aspects of evidence gathering that affect perception of credibility of evaluation results:

- Stakeholders are more likely to accept the conclusions and recommendations of the evaluation when they have been actively involved in defining and gathering data that they find credible. Health care managers and providers will increase their sense of responsibility in the services they provide and will be able to assess their own accomplishments.
- The number of measurements used should be limited. If not, the whole data collection process gets too burdensome. However, multiple indicators are usually needed for tracking the implementation and effectiveness of a programme. Using the logic model to define a spectrum of indicators can be very useful. For cervical cancer screening, for example, the model presented in Figure 10.3 can be used to define indicators such as the compliance to screening (of the target age group), compliance to diagnosis and treatment (of women with abnormal Pap smears), as well as the time it takes women to go through each step of the process.
- Performance indicators should be well defined and analysed within the context of the programme. For example, a reduction in the mortality of cervical cancer may be also influenced by improved standards of living among at risk women or by improved access to treatment of early invasive cancers, and not only to the screening programme.
- Multiple sources of information, which include different perspectives, enhance the credibility of the evaluation. The criteria used for selecting sources should be stated clearly so users are aware of the limitations and the interpretation of the information can be done correctly.
- Quality, quantity, and logistics for gathering the evidence will also affect the credibility of the evaluation. Quality refers to the appropriateness and integrity of the information used. Well-defined indicators enable easier collection of quality data. Quantity of the information should be established in advance. It affects the potential confidence level and partly determines whether the evaluation will have sufficient power to detect effects. The procedures for gathering the evidence must be easy and the timeframe short enough so that the data collection can be repeated frequently to allow for trend changes over time without being too much of a burden on the system.

What standards (type or level of performance) must be reached for the national cancer control programme to be considered successful?

The standards are values set by stakeholders, and these reflect the principles of a national cancer control programme as well as the expected results in both the processes and the outcomes. Regarding the principles of a national cancer control programme described in Chapter 10, standards should be developed to assess how the implementation of the national cancer control programme is corresponding with those principles. In the case of process and outcome measures, they should be feasible and adjusted to the context of the programme as well as to its stage of development.

Regarding outcome measures, the reduction in the incidence of tobacco-related cancers will take over 20 years, and a screening programme may take at least 10 years to show reduction in mortality rates. Thus, in the first years of development of a national cancer control programme the emphasis should be on process measures and short-term outcome measures. It should be taken into consideration that within political circles, there may be unrealistic expectations concerning the time needed to achieve the programme's long-term objectives. Stakeholders may have different ideas about programme goals and objectives. It should be pointed out that, despite general recognition in the 1960s that cigarette smoking was a cause of lung cancer, it was the end of the 1980s before the resulting control measures began to have an appreciable impact on lung cancer mortality in North America and the United Kingdom. Similarly, even if a population shows adequate compliance with screening, it may be more than 10 years before mortality from a particular form of cancer begins to decline. Hence the short-term emphasis (that is, within the first 5 years) should be on process measures that confirm initially that the relevant component of the programme is in place. These should be followed with measures that will indicate whether there has been sufficient uptake of the activity for there to be an impact on outcome measures in the medium term (within 10 years) and the long term (15–20 years).

What conclusions regarding a national cancer control programme performance are justified by comparing available evidence to the standards?

Conclusions of the evaluation can be justified by judging the evidence gathered against values or standards set by stakeholders. This allows the identification of gaps between present programme performance and desired performance and determination of which kinds of actions must be implemented to bridge those gaps. Usually the gaps are due to lack of resources; but even more importantly, they are often due to improper management, inefficient use of limited resources, improper translation of the evidence into practice, lack of motivation, weaknesses in skills and knowledge of healthcare providers; and limited participation of consumers in the decision-making process.

How will lessons learnt from the results of the evaluation be used to improving national cancer control programme performance?

Effort is needed to ensure that the evaluation results are disseminated and appropriately used in the decision-making process.

The following are critical elements for ensuring appropriate use of an evaluation.

- evaluation recommendations must be ready when needed; thus timeliness is essential;
- reporting techniques must suit the users and be adapted to different audiences;
- a detailed plan of action for improving performance must be elaborated with the participation of primary users of the evaluation and other relevant stakeholders;
- follow up is needed to ensure consistency between findings and subsequent actions.

Chapter 11 describes a model for changing established practices of health care providers in the workplace that can be useful to apply if substantial reorganization is needed to improve the programme's performance.

Specific considerations regarding outcome evaluation of the different programme components of prevention, early detection, treatment and palliative care are discussed below.

Evaluation of prevention

The major determinants of the risk of cancer are clearly related to individual lifestyle (for example, tobacco usage and diet) and environment factors (for example, solar radiation). At the population level, therefore, cancer patterns depend on the prevalence of such exposures, and the risk each one poses to the individual. The WHO stepwise approach to surveillance (STEPS), described in Chapter 9, provides a methodology for measuring the key risk factors for noncommunicable diseases, including cancer. The risk factors for cancer monitored in the STEPS surveillance mechanism include:

- tobacco use;
- alcohol;
- nutrition;
- physical inactivity; and
- obesity.

The first step of this methodology involves the use of standardized questionnaires. The second step comprises physical measurements. The third step includes biochemical measurements. At each step the core information can be expanded, to the extent resources permit.

In addition to the above mentioned risk factors, several infections are important causes of cancer. These include:
- hepatitis B and C viruses, important causes of liver cancer;
- human papillomavirus (HPV), a major cause of cancer of the cervix;
- HIV infection, a major cause of sarcoma and non-Hodgkin lymphoma.

Prevalence surveys are available for hepatitis B and C, HIV and HPV infections.

Lastly, the exposure of inadequately protected workers to carcinogenic chemicals should be evaluated. Special government departments dealing with occupational hazards usually monitor this.

Cancer control by prevention has a long timescale, often 15-20 years. Usually, evaluation is based upon time trends in incidence of cancer, to see whether the desired effect is being achieved. For cancers with a poor, or unchanging survival, mortality rates may be used for the same purpose. Examples are the monitoring of the incidence of tobacco-related cancer in response to tobacco control programmes or, in the longer term, of liver cancer following hepatitis vaccination. Occasionally, when implementation has been confined to one area, comparisons of the changes in the intervention area with the situation in 'control' areas may be possible.

Evaluation of early detection

Outcome evaluation of early detection programmes depends upon measuring whether their ultimate objective has been achieved. Thus, screening for cervical cancer aims to reduce incidence of invasive cancer. This is also the aim of oral cancer detection programmes. Other screening programmes, which aim to detect invasive cancers early (for example, breast), do not reduce incidence. Incidence may increase initially, as such programmes bring forward the diagnosis date of pre-existing but undiagnosed cancers. The objective in this case is to decrease mortality.

Time trend studies may examine trends in incidence in relation to screening activity. For instance, the population-based registries in the Nordic countries provided data on time trends in incidence of cervical cancer in relation to screening (Hakama, 1982). The fall in incidence was closely related to the coverage offered by the organized mass screening programmes. The introduction of screening was followed by an apparent increase in incidence as prevalent sub-clinical cases were detected, before a fall was observed. Other similar studies have compared the change in incidence of cervical cancer with the registration (detection) rate of carcinoma *in situ* in different geographical areas.

When the records of the screening programme can be linked with those of a population-based cancer registry, it is possible to compare the risk of cancer in those screened and those not screened. It is also possible to estimate the incidence of cancer at different intervals (within 1 year, 1–2 years, and so on.) after a negative screening test, as a fraction of the "expected" incidence without screening. This rate of "interval cancers" is a very useful indicator of the sensitivity of the programme (Day, Williams, Khaw, 1989)

Case-control studies have also been widely used to evaluate early detection programmes. The principle is to study the past history of screening in cases of cancer, and compare this with an appropriate control group (Prorok, 1984). This approach has been used, for example, in auditing cervical cancer screening programmes (Sasieni, Cuzick, Lynch, 1996). Cohort studies and case-control studies of screening must, however be interpreted with care, as they cannot exclude selection bias, and they measure the effect of choosing to be screened. For cancer of the cervix, people who chose to be screened are often at lower risk of the disease, even without the test (selection bias).

Although earlier detection, as shown by 'intermediate endpoints', such as the size or stage of cancers detected, as recorded by the registry, is essential if a screening programme is to be successful in reducing mortality, it is no guarantee that it will do so. Intermediate endpoints may appear to improve, even though mortality does not.

Thus, only when a screening programme is known to be effective should intermediate endpoints be used to monitor it. Suitable monitoring statistics from cancer registries are:

- the incidence of interval cancers;
- the size and stage distribution of cancers detected by screening (compared to the expected distribution);
- the incidence rate of advanced cancers, compared with the period pre-screening (or an unscreened comparison group).

These important indicators, provided by population-based registries, are now widely used to monitor the effectiveness of breast cancer screening programmes.

Changes in the stage at which cancer of the cervix, breast, and mouth is diagnosed should be evaluated at cancer treatment centres. Evaluation of population coverage in screening programmes should concentrate particularly on coverage of target age groups, rural areas, and low socioeconomic groups. The proportion of people with abnormalities revealed in screening tests who subsequently obtain appropriate diagnosis and treatment should be determined, as should the proportion of all cases of particular cancers that were diagnosed by screening. The technical quality of screening tests and of the facilities that undertake them should also be carefully monitored.

With a view to future expansion of the screening programme by coverage of a wider age range or increase in the frequency of screening, the monitoring of staff development and training processes is essential.

Evaluation of treatment

Many cancer registries aim to follow up their cases, in order to produce survival statistics. Follow up is active (contacting the patient or their relatives), or by matching death certificates against cancer notifications and assuming that unmatched cases are still alive.

Survival following a diagnosis of cancer is used to evaluate the impact of the extent to which new or improved cancer treatments are incorporated in clinical practice. Such measures at the population level are quite different from the survival rates reported by studies of selected case series or clinical trials. For instance, the advances made in clinical trial settings in the treatment of childhood cancers, Hodgkin disease and testicular tumours, have already been widely implemented in the community in many industrialized countries, and the population-based survival from these cancers has shown a significant increase over the last three decades.

Comparisons of cancer survival rates are increasingly used to compare the effectiveness of cancer treatment in different populations (including within the same country, for example by region, or by social class). This requires careful standardization of the registry methods (definition of incident cases, date of diagnosis, method of follow up). Comparisons also mean that other parameters, such as stage distribution, are known, since these greatly influence the success of treatment.

Cancer registries are increasingly being used to look at patterns of care received by cancer patients, and whether these meet pre-set criteria, with a view to improving the services provided. Thus, for example, it may be possible to see what proportion of patients appear to wait a long time between diagnosis and treatment, or receive treatment in hospitals not adapted to their needs.

Evaluation of palliative care

Evaluating the outcome of palliative care will usually require setting up special mechanisms to assess quality of life. Special studies may be conducted among patients, their families and healthcare providers considering the various dimensions of quality of life: pain relief and other symptom control, functionality, psychosocial and spiritual well-being, family and medical interaction, financial issues, and so on. There are several quality-of-life instruments available in the literature but very few have been validated within palliative care populations. Further development of these tools is needed, especially for palliative care populations from different cultural and socioeconomic settings.

Focusing on Priorities

A LL COUNTRIES should endeavour to implement national cancer control programmes, with a view to reducing cancer incidence and mortality, improving quality of life, and reducing cancer risk factors.

What can actually be implemented and achieved depends on a variety of factors, including the resources available. Chapter 13 outlines the priority actions that countries should undertake, according to their level of resources.

PRIORITIES FOR VARIOUS RESOURCE LEVELS

13

All countries should aim to implement a national cancer control programme within a comprehensive, systemic framework. The recommendations for minimum essential actions by national cancer control programmes, in countries with different levels of resources, are summarized in Table 13.1. This is the best way to effectively reduce cancer incidence and mortality, improve survival and quality of life, and reduce cancer risk factors by making the most efficient use of resources. Special attention should be given to the training of health care workers at the different levels of care. The level of complexity of the training will depend on the role each worker plays. Health care workers should be trained in basic skills that allow them to integrate palliative care, prevention and early detection activities into their daily work.

Moreover, all countries should establish core surveillance and information systems that allow them to monitor and evaluate epidemiological and programmatic data, and to use this data as a basis for appropriate decision-making.

Countries with low to medium levels of resources should consider addressing key priorities in a demonstration area. Each priority can be approached in a stepwise manner allowing for a systematic progression and expansion, both in terms of programme content and in geographical scope. It is also important to ensure the use of appropriate technology that is cost-effective and sustainable in situations where resources are constrained.

For countries with low levels of resources, where the majority of patients are currently diagnosed in advanced stages, low-cost and effective palliative care may constitute a powerful entry point, progressively leading to a more comprehensive approach that includes early diagnosis and primary prevention.

Countries with high levels of resources can afford full implementation of evidence-based strategies within the framework of a national cancer control programme. A review of current resource allocation, followed by an adjustment of strategies to allow more efficient and effective use of resources, releases funds that can then be directed to improving weak areas in the cancer field or provide support for less affluent countries.

Table 13.1 Priority actions for national cancer control programmes, according to lèvel of resources

Component	All countries	Scenario A: Low level of resources	Scenario B: Medium level of resources	Scenario C: High level of resources
National cancer control programme	• Develop a national cancer control programme to ensure effective, efficient and equitable use of existing resources • Establish a core surveillance mechanism to monitor and evaluate outcomes as well as processes • Develop education and continuous training for health care workers	• Consider the implementation of one or two key priorities in a demonstration area with a stepwise approach • Consider palliative care as an entry point to a more comprehensive approach • Use appropriate technologies that are effective and sustainable in this type of setting	• When initiating or formulating a cancer control programme, consider implementation of a comprehensive approach in a demonstration area using a stepwise methodology • Use appropriate technologies that are effective and sustainable in this type of setting	• Full, nationwide implementation of evidence-based strategies guaranteeing effectiveness, efficiency, and accessibility • Implement a comprehensive surveillance system, tracking all programme components and results • Provide support for less affluent countries
Prevention	• Implement integrated health promotion and prevention strategies for noncommunicable diseases that include legislative/regulatory and environmental measures as well as education for the general public, targeted communities and individuals • Control tobacco use, and address alcohol use, unhealthy diet, physical activity and sexual and reproductive factors • Promote policy to minimize occupational-related cancers and known environmental carcinogens • Promote avoidance of unnecessary exposure to sunlight in high risk populations	• Focus on areas where there are great needs and potential for success • Ensure that priority prevention strategics arc targeted to those groups that are influential and can spearhead the process (e.g., policy-makers, and teachers) • In areas endemic for liver cancer, integrate HBV with other vaccination programmes	• Develop integrated clinical preventive services for counselling on risk factors in primary health care settings, schools and workplaces • Develop model community programmes for an integrated approach to prevention of noncommunicable diseases	• Strengthen comprehensive evidence-based health promotion and prevention programmes and ensure nationwide implementation in collaboration with other sectors • Establish routine monitoring of ultraviolet radiation levels if the risk of skin cancer is high
Early diagnosis	• Promote early diagnosis through awareness of early signs and symptoms of detectable and curable tumours that have high prevalence in the community, such as breast and cervical cancer • Ensure proper diagnostic and treatment services are available for the detected cases • Provide education and continuous training to target populations and health care providers	• Use low cost and effective community approaches to promote, in a first phase, early diagnosis of one or two priority detectable tumours in a pilot area with relatively good access to diagnosis and treatment	• Use low cost and effective community approaches to promote early diagnosis of all priority detectable tumours	• Use comprehensive nationwide promotion strategies for early diagnosis of all highly prevalent detectable tumours
Screening	• Implement screening for cancers of the breast and cervix where incidence justifies such action and the necessary resources are available	• If there is already infrastructure for cervical cytology screening, provide high coverage of effective and efficient cytology screening for women aged 35 to 40 years once in their lifetime or, if more resources are available, every 10 years for women aged 30 to 60 years	• Provide national coverage cytology screening for cervical cancer at 5 year intervals to women aged 30 to 60 years	• Effective and efficient national screening for cervical cancer (cytology) of women over 30 years old and breast cancer screening (mammography) of women over 50 years of age
Curative therapy	• Ensure accessibility of effective diagnostic and treatment services • Promote national minimum essential standards for disease staging and treatment • Establish management guidelines for treatment services, essential drugs list, and continuous training • Avoid performing curative therapy when cancer is incurable and patients should be offered palliative care instead	• Organize diagnosis and treatment services giving priority to early detectable tumours	• Organize diagnosis and treatment services, giving priority to early detectable tumours or to those with high potential of curability	• Reinforce the network of comprehensive cancer treatment centres that are active for clinical training and research and give special support to the ones acting as national and international reference centres
Pain relief and palliative care	• Implement comprehensive palliative care that provides pain relief, other symptom control, and psychosocial and spiritual support • Promote national minimum standards for management of pain and palliative care • Ensure availability and accessibility of opioids, especially oral morphine • Provide education and training for carers and public	• Ensure that minimum standards for pain relief and palliative care are progressively adopted by all levels of care in targeted areas and that there is high coverage of patients through services provided mainly by home-based care	• Ensure that minimum standards for pain relief and palliative care are progressively adopted by all levels of care and nationwide there is rising coverage of patients through services provided by primary health care clinics and home-based care	• Ensure that national pain relief and palliative care guidelines are adopted by all levels of care and nationwide there is high coverage of patients through a variety of options, including home-based care

168

PRIORITY PREVENTION ACTIONS FOR VARIOUS RESOURCE LEVELS

All countries should give priority to implementing integrated health promotion and prevention strategies for noncommunicable diseases that are consistent with the present and projected epidemiological situation. As a minimum, these interventions should include tobacco prevention and control, reduction of alcohol use, promotion of a healthy diet and physical activity, and education about sexual and reproductive factors.

Furthermore, all countries should establish policies aimed at minimizing occupationally-related cancers, and legislate to control known environmental carcinogenic agents. Strategies should include legislation and regulation, environmental measures, and education at community, school and individual levels.

Avoidance of unnecessary exposure to sunlight should be recommended, particularly in high-risk populations.

Low-resource countries should focus on areas where there are not only great needs, but also the potential for success. They should ensure that priority prevention strategies are targeted to those groups that are influential and can spearhead the whole process, such as policy-makers, health workers, and teachers. In areas with a high prevalence of cancers induced by biological agents, special measures should be developed to combat the infections concerned, for example, schistosomiasis and hepatitis B. In areas endemic for liver cancer, HBV vaccination should be integrated with other vaccination programmes.

Countries with medium levels of resources should consider developing clinical services for brief, effective counselling on tobacco cessation and other cancer risk factors and strengthening education for healthy lifestyles. These activities should take place in primary health care settings, schools and workplaces. Medium-resource countries should also consider developing model community programmes for an integrated approach to the prevention of noncommunicable diseases.

Countries with high levels of resources should implement comprehensive, evidence-based health promotion and prevention programmes, and ensure nationwide implementation of these programmes in collaboration with other sectors. Routine monitoring of ultraviolet radiation levels should be established if the risk of skin cancer is high.

RECOMMENDED EARLY DETECTION POLICIES FOR VARIOUS RESOURCE LEVELS

Early Diagnosis (already symptomatic populations)

As part of a national cancer control programme, all countries should promote awareness of the warning signs for those cancers that display signs and symptoms early in the evolution of the disease. The public should be educated about the changes to watch for, and what to do if they notice these signs. Health workers should be trained to recognize early cancer cases, and refer them rapidly to places where the disease can be diagnosed and treated. Cancer sites amenable to early diagnosis include: oral cavity, larynx, colorectum, skin, breast, cervix, urinary bladder, and prostate.

In low-resource settings, low cost and effective community approaches should be used in the first phase to promote early diagnosis of one or two priority detectable tumours. This approach should be adopted initially in a pilot area with relatively good access to diagnosis and treatment.

Countries with medium levels of resources should use low-cost and effective community approaches to promote early diagnosis of all priority detectable tumours.

Countries with high levels of resources should use comprehensive nationwide promotion strategies for early diagnosis of all highly prevalent, detectable tumours.

Screening (asymptomatic populations)

Where level of incidence of the cancer justify it, and the necessary resources can be made available, screening for cancers of the breast and cervix is recommended. This is feasible mainly in medium- and high-resource level countries. Screening for other cancer sites must be regarded as experimental and cannot be recommended at present as public health policy. All countries implementing screening policies should consider the programmatic factors that determine whether or not the programmes achieve effectiveness and efficiency.

In low-resource countries, if there is already infrastructure for cervical cytology screening, the recommendation is to provide high coverage of effective and efficient cytology screening for women 35–40 years old once in their lifetime or, if more resources are available, every 10 years for women 30–60 years old.

Low-income countries that do not have screening facilities should be discouraged from initiating cytology screening. They should wait until the cost-effectiveness of a low cost approach (VIA) is demonstrated.

Countries with medium levels of resources should aim to provide national coverage by cytology screening for cervical cancer at 5-year intervals to women 30–60 years old.

Countries with high levels of resources should reinforce and improve the performance of national screening for cervical cancer and breast cancer if those cancers are common.

PRIORITY ACTIONS FOR CANCER TREATMENT ACCORDING TO RESOURCE LEVELS

All countries should ensure the accessibility and effectiveness of diagnosis and treatment services by establishing evidence-based clinical and management guidelines, an essential drugs list, good referral, follow-up and evaluation systems, and continuous training of the different health professionals involved. Furthermore, guidelines should emphasize the avoidance of offering curative therapy when cancer is incurable, and patients should be offered palliative care instead.

Countries with low or medium levels of resources should organize diagnosis and treatment services to give priority to common, early detectable tumours, or to those with high potential for cure.

Countries with a high level of resources should reinforce the development of comprehensive cancer treatment and palliative care centres that are especially active for clinical training and research, and that can act as reference centres within the country as well as at the international level.

PRIORITY ACTIONS FOR PALLIATIVE CARE ACCORDING TO RESOURCE LEVELS

All countries should implement comprehensive palliative care programmes with the purpose of improving the quality of life of the majority of patients with cancer, or other life-threatening conditions, and their families. These programmes should provide pain relief, other symptom control, and psychosocial and spiritual support. All countries should promote awareness among the public and health professionals that cancer pain can be avoided, and should ensure the availability of oral morphine in all healthcare settings.

In low-resource settings it is important to ensure that minimum standards for pain relief and palliative care are progressively adopted at all levels of care in targeted areas, and that there is high coverage of patients through services provided mainly by home-based care. Home-based care is generally the best way of achieving good quality care and coverage in countries with strong family support and poor health infrastructure.

Countries with medium levels of resources should ensure that minimum standards for cancer pain relief and palliative care are progressively adopted at all levels of care, and that, nationwide, there is increasing coverage of patients through services provided by health care workers and home-based care.

Meeting participants

The valuable contributions made by the following participants at major meetings on the theme of this monograph are gratefully acknowledged:

WHO Working Group on National Cancer Control Programmes (Geneva, 25–29 November 1991)

Mr W. A. Adair, Cancer 2000, Toronto, Canada

Dr K. Anantha, Kidwai Memorial Institute of Oncology, Bangalore, India

Dr B. Armstrong, International Agency for Research on Cancer, Lyon, France

Dr H. Barnum, World Bank, Washington, DC, USA

Dr J. M. Borras, Department of Health and Social Security, Government of Catalonia, Barcelona, Spain

Dr L. Breslow, Center for Health Promotion/Disease Prevention, School of Public Health, Los Angeles, CA, USA

Dr R. Camacho, National Institute of Cancer and Radiobiology, Havana, Cuba

Dr H. Danielsson, Cancer and Palliative Care, World Health Organization, Geneva, Switzerland

Dr L. Fernandez, National Institute of Cancer and Radiobiology, Havana, Cuba

Dr J. A. M. Gray, Oxfordshire Department of Public Health, Headington, England

Dr J. D. F. Habbema, Department of Public Health and Social Medicine, Erasmus University, Rotterdam, Netherlands

Dr T. Hakulinen, Finnish Cancer Registry, Institute for Statistical and Epidemiological Cancer Research, Helsinki, Finland

Dr R. C. Hickey, International Union Against Cancer, Geneva, Switzerland

Dr M. K. M. Ismail, Tanta Cancer Institute, Cairo, Egypt

Dr N. A. Jafarey, College of Physicians and Surgeons, Karachi, Pakistan

Dr L. M. Jerry, Alberta Cancer Program, Calgary, Canada

Dr C. F. Kiire, WHO Regional Office for Africa, Brazzaville, Congo

Dr L. Komarova, Cancer Research Centre, Moscow, Russian Federation

Dr V. Koroltchouk, Cancer and Palliative Care, World Health Organization, Geneva, Switzerland

Dr G. Llanos, WHO Regional Office for the Americas, Washington, DC, USA

Dr A. Lopez, Global Health Situation Assessment and Projection, World Health Organization, Geneva, Switzerland

Dr U. Luthra, Indian Council for Medical Research, New Delhi, India

Dr J. Magrath, National Cancer Institute, Bethesda, MD, USA

Dr R. Margolese, Jewish General Hospital, Montreal, Canada

Dr A. Mbakop, University of Yaoundeç, Yaoundeç, Cameroon

Dr T. R. Möller, Southern Swedish Regional Tumour Registry, University Hospital, Lund, Sweden

Dr K. Nair, Regional Cancer Centre, Trivandrum, India

Dr E. J. Ospina, Pathology Clinic Palermo, Bogota, Colombia

Dr A. Roxas, Department of Health, Philippine Cancer Control Programme, Manila, Philippines

Dr V. Sagaidak, Division of Cancer Control, Cancer Research Centre, Moscow, Russian Federation

Dr H. Sell, WHO Regional Office for South–East Asia, New Delhi, India

Dr C. Sepulveda, Ministry of Health, Santiago, Chile

Dr T. F. Solanke, National Headquarters of Cancer Registries in Nigeria, University College Hospital, Ibadan, Nigeria

Dr R. Sweet, Commission of the European Communities, Brussels, Belgium

Dr Tan Chor–Hiang, Ministry of Health, Singapore

Dr N. Trapeznikov, Cancer Research Centre, Moscow, Russian Federation

Ms M. Truax, Nursing, World Health Organization, Geneva, Switzerland

Mr A. J. Turnbull, International Union Against Cancer, Geneva, Switzerland

Dr M. H. Wahdan, WHO Regional Office for the Eastern Mediterranean, Alexandria, Egypt

Dr L. Waldstrom, Oncological Centre for Southern Sweden, University Hospital, Lund, Sweden

Dr B. Wasisto, Ministry of Health, Jakarta, Indonesia

Dr F. Zadra, European School of Oncology, Milan, Italy

Dr S. H. M. Zaidi, Jannah Postgraduate Medical Centre, Karachi, Pakistan

WHO Working Group on National Cancer Control Programmes
(Banff, 26 September–1 October 1993)

Dr M. Al–Jarallah, Kuwait Cancer Control Centre, Kuwait

Dr H. G. Al–Jazzaf, Kuwait Cancer Control Centre, Kuwait

Dr A. Alwan, WHO Regional Office for the Eastern Mediterranean, Alexandria, Egypt

Dr C. Atkinson, Christchurch Hospital, Christchurch, New Zealand

Dr J. Bauer, Charles University, Prague, Czech Republic

Mr H. Barnum, World Bank, Washington, DC, USA

Dr C. Bratti, Health Directorate, San Josée, Costa Rica

Dr R. Calderon–Saniz, Ministry of Social Welfare and Public Health, La Paz, Bolivia

Dr R. Camacho Rodriguez, National Institute of Cancer and Radiobiology, Havana, Cuba

Ms S. Dahl, Ministry of Health, Wellington, New Zealand

Mr T. K. Das, Ministry of Health and Family Welfare, New Delhi, India

Dr T. D. Devaraj, National Cancer Society of Malaysia, Penang, Malaysia

Dr J. Fins, Cornell Medical Center, New York, NY, USA

Mr W. Foster, Tom Baker Cancer Centre, Calgary, Alberta, Canada

Dr P. Géher, Ministry of Welfare, Budapest, Hungary

Professor M. A. Hai, Cancer Institute and Research Hospital, Mohakhali, Dhaka, Bangladesh

Mrs E. Henry, New South Wales Cancer Council, Sydney, New South Wales, Australia

Dr E. Hill, Department of Health, London, England

Dr L. E. Holm, National Institute of Public Health, Stockholm, Sweden

Dr M. A. Jaffer, Ministry of Health, Muscat, Oman

Dr M. Jerry, WHO Collaborating Centre for Cancer Control, Tom Baker Cancer Centre, Calgary, Alberta, Canada

Dr E. A. R. Kaegi, National Cancer Institute of Canada, Toronto, Ontario, Canada

Dr M. Kasler, National Institute of Oncology, Budapest, Hungary

Dr V. Koroltchouk, Cancer and Palliative Care, World Health Organization, Geneva, Switzerland

Dr R. Lappi, National Research and Development Centre, Helsinki, Finland

Dr J. M. Larranaga, Health Ministry, Montevideo, Uruguay

Dr M. Laugesen, Public Health Commission, Wellington, New Zealand

Dr A. Legaspi, Juarez Hospital, Cuahulemo, Mexico

Dr F. Li, Laboratory Centre for Disease Control, Health Canada, Ottawa, Ontario, Canada

Dr T. J. Liebenberg, Cancer Association of South Africa, Johannesburg, South Africa

Dr R. R. Love, University of Wisconsin, Madison, WI, USA

Dr N. MacDonald, University of Alberta, Edmonton, Alberta, Canada

Dr S. S. Manraj, Central Health Laboratory, Quatre–Bornes, Mauritius

Dr B. Mashbadrakh, National Centre of Oncology, Ulaanbaatar, Mongolia

Dr B. Mathew, Regional Cancer Centre, Trivandrum, India

Ms P. Messervy, Ministry of Health, Wellington, New Zealand

Ms M. B. Msika, Ministry of Health and Child Welfare, Harare, Zimbabwe

Dr H. Mustun, Victoria Hospital, Candos, Mauritius

Dr M. K. Nair, Regional Cancer Centre, Trivandrum, India

Dr J. Ospina, International Union Against Cancer, Santa Feª de Bogota•, Colombia

Dr S. Puribhat, National Cancer Institute, Bangkok, Thailand

Dr B. Randeniya, Cancer Institute, Maharagama, Sri Lanka

Dr A. Roxas, Philippines Cancer Control Program, Manila, Philippines

Dr R. Sanson–Fisher, New South Wales Cancer Council, Wallsend, New South Wales, Australia

Dr H. Schipper, St Boniface General Hospital Research Centre, Winnipeg, Manitoba, Canada

Dr C. Sepulveda, Ministry of Health, Santiago, Chile

Dr T. F. Solanke, National Headquarters of Cancer Registries in Nigeria, Ibadan, Nigeria

Dr S. Stachenko, Health Canada, Ottawa, Ontario, Canada

Dr H. Storm, Danish Cancer Society, Division of Cancer Epidemiology, Copenhagen, Denmark

Dr G. Stuart, Tom Baker Cancer Centre, Calgary, Alberta, Canada

Dr F.C. M. Sungani, National Cancer Committee, Blantyre, Malawi

Dr Tan Chor–Hiang, Ministry of Health, Singapore

Dr E. W. Trevelyan, Harvard School of Public Health, Boston, MA, USA

Dr B. B. Vaidya, B.P. Koirala Memorial Cancer Hospital, Kathmandu, Nepal

Dr Z. Zain, Ministry of Health, Kuala Lumpur, Malaysia

Dr M. P. Zakelj, Institute of Oncology, Ljubljana, Slovenia

WHO Meeting on National Cancer Control Programmes: Review of progress made with special emphasis on developing countries, held in WHO (Geneva, 5–8 December 2000)

Dr A. Alwan, Management of Noncommunicable Diseases Department, WHO

Dr A. Al–Asfour, Kuwait Cancer Center, Kuwait

Dr N. Al–Hamdan, National Cancer Registry, Riyadh, Saudi Arabia

Dr M. Belhocine, AFRO, WHO

Dr C. Boshi–Pinto, Burden of Disease Department, WHO

Dr K. A. Dinshaw, Tata Memorial Centre, Mumbai, India

Dr N. B. Duc, National Cancer Institute, Hanoi, Vietnam

Dr M. Borok, University of Zimbabwe, Harare, Zimbabwe

Dr A. S. Doh, University of Yaounde, Yaounde, Cameroon

Dr S. Fonn, Women's Health Project, Johannesburg, South Africa

Professor V. Grabauskas, Kaunas University of Medicine, Kaunas, Lithuania

Dr D. Hunter, Harvard School of Public Health, Boston, USA

Dr O. Khatib, EMRO, WHO

Dr J. Kligerman, Braz ilian National Cancer Institute, Rio de Janeiro, Brazil

Dr S. Kvinnsland, Norwegian Cancer Society, Oslo, Norway

Dr J. Leowski, SEARO, WHO

Dr V. Levin, International Atomic Energy Agency, Vienna, Austria

Ms N. Macklai, Tobacco Free Initiative, WHO

Dr N. MacDonald, Clinical Research Institute of Montreal, Montreal, Canada

Dr A. Merriman, Hospice Uganda, Kampala, Uganda

Dr A. B. Miller, Deutsches Krebsforschungszentrum, Heidelberg, Germany

Mrs I. Motara, International Union Against Cancer, Geneva, Switzerland

Dr K. Nair, Regional Cancer Institute, Thiruvanthapuram, India

Dr T. Ngoma, Ocean Road Cancer Institute, Dar es Salaam, United Republic of Tanzania

Dr C. Olweny, St Boniface general Hospital, Winnipeg, Canada

Dr D. M. Parkin, IARC, Lyon, France

Dr E. Papulin, Disability and Rehabilitation, WHO

Dr S. Robles, PAHO, WHO

Dr H. Sancho–Garnier, Montpelier, France

Dr R. Sankaranarayanan, IARC, Lyon, France

Dr C. Sepulveda, Cancer Control Programme, WHO

DR A. Shatchkute, EURO, WHO

Dr K. Stanley, Cancer Control Programme, WHO

Dr J. Sternsward, Svedala, Sweden

Dr K. Strong, Management of Noncommunicable Diseases Department, WHO

Dr R. G. Twycross, The Churchill Hospital, Oxford, United Kingdom

Professor V. Ventafridda, Instituto Europeo di Oncologia, Milan, Italy

Dr D. Yach, Noncommunicable Diseases and Mental Health, WHO

REFERENCES

Abed J Reilly B Butler MO et al. Developing a framework for comprehensive cancer prevention and control in the United States: an initiative of the Centers for Disease Control and Prevention. *Journal of Public Health Management Practice* 6:67–78.

American Joint Committee on Cancer (1997) *AJCC Cancer Staging Manual.* 5th ed, Philadelphia, PA, Lippincott–Raven Publishers.

American Medical Association. Institute for Ethics (1999) *EPEC: education for physicians on end–of–life care.* Chicago,III: American Medical Association: EPEC Project, The Robert Wood Johnson Foundation.

Armstrong BK. (1992) The role of the cancer registry in cancer control. *Cancer Causes and Control,* 3:569–579.

Artvinli M, Baris Y. (1979) Malignant mesothelioma in a small village in the Anatolian region of Turkey: an epidemiologic study. *Journal of the National Cancer Institute,* 63:17–22.

Barrows HS, Tamblyn RM. (1980) *Problem–based learning: an approach to medical education.* New York, Springer Publishing Company.

Berrino F et al., eds. (1999) *Survival of Cancer Patients in Europe: the EUROCARE–2 Study.* Lyon, IARC Scientific Publications No. 151.

Bonita et al. (2001) *Surveillance of risk factors for noncommunicable diseases: The WHO STEPwise approach.* Geneva, WHO.

Brazil K, (1999) A framework for developing evaluation capacity in health care settings. *International Journal of Health Care Quality Assurance Incorporating Leadership in Health Services,* 12:vi–xi.

Brown ML, Hodgson TA, Rice DP. (1996) Economic impact of cancer in the United States. In: Schottenfeld D, Fraumeni JF Jr., eds. *Cancer Epidemiology and Prevention,* 2nd ed. New York, Oxford University Press, 255–266.

Buckman R. (1996) Talking to patients about cancer. *British Medical Journal,* 313: 699–700.

Canadian Council on Health Services Accreditation (1996) *A guide to the development and use of performance indicators.* Ottawa, Canadian Council on Health Services Accreditation.

Centano–Cortes C, Nunez–Olarte JM. (1994) Questioning diagnosis disclosure in terminal cancer patients: a prospective study evaluating patient responses. *Journal of Cancer Education,* 8: 39–44.

Centers for Disease Control and Prevention (1999) Framework for program evaluation in public health. MMWR 48 (No. RR–11)

Committee on Environmental Epidemiology (1991). *Hazardous Waste Sites.* Washington, DC, National Academy Press.

Day NE, Williams DR, Khaw KT. (1989) Breast cancer screening programmes: the development of a monitoring and evaluation system. *British Journal of Cancer,* 59: 954–958.

Doll R, Peto R. (1981) The causes of cancer: quantitative estimates of avoidable risks of cancer in the United States today. *Journal of the National Cancer Institute,* 66:1191–1308.

Donabedian A (1980) *Explorations in quality assessment and monitoring.* Ann Arbor, Michigan, Health Administration Press.

Dunlop RJ, Campbell CW. (2000) Cytokines and advanced cancer. *Journal of Pain and Symptom Management.* 20: 214–232.

Eddy D. (1986) Setting priorities for cancer control programs. *Journal of the National Cancer Institute,* 76:187–199.

EPIC Investigators (2002, In press) Fruit and vegetables and colorectal cancer. In: Riboli E, Lambert R eds. *Nutrition and life style: opportunities for cancer prevention.* Lyon. IARC Scientific Publication No 156 IARC Press.

Epping–Jordan JE et al. (1999) Psychological adjustment in breast cancer: Processes of emotional distress. *Health Psychology,* 18: 315–326.

Faulkner A, et al. (1995) Improving the skills of doctors in giving distressing information. *Medical Education* 29: 303–7.

Faulkner A, Peace G, O'Keeffe C. (1993) Cancer care: future imperfect. *Nursing Times,* 89: 40–3.

Ferlay J et al. (2000) GLOBOCAN 2000: *Cancer Incidence Mortality and Prevalence Worldwide.* Lyon. IARC CancerBase No. 5.

Fonn S. (2001) Prevalence data and costing considerations in service planning – the case of cervical cancer. In: Sundari Ravindran TK eds. *Transforming Health Systems: Gender and Rights in Reproductive Health.* Geneva, WHO.

Gastrin G et al. (1994) Incidence and mortality from breast cancer in the Mama program for breast screening in Finland, 1973 – 1986. *Cancer,* 73:2168–2174.

Global Forum for Health Research (2000) *Global Forum for Health Research: an overview.* Geneva, WHO.

Gray MJA (2001) *Evidence Based Health Care,* 2nd Ed. London, Churchill Livingstone.

Greenwald P, Kramer BS, Weed DL. (1995) *Cancer prevention and control.* New York. Marcel Dekker Inc.

Greenwald P, Sondik EJ, Young JL. (1986) Emerging roles for cancer registries in cancer control. *Yale Journal of Biology and Medicine* 59: 561–566

Gupta PC. (1996) Survey of sociodemographic characteristics of tobacco use among 99,598 individuals in Bombay, India using handheld computers. *Tobacco Control,* 5: 114–120.

Hakama M. (1982) Trends in the Incidence of Cervical Cancer in the Nordic Countries. In: Magnus K, ed. *Trends in cancer incidence*. Washington, DC, Hemisphere.

Hakama M et al. (1975) Incidence, mortality or prevalence as indicators of the cancer problem. *Cancer,* 36:2227–31.

Hakama M et al. (1985) Evaluation of screening programmes for gynaecological cancer. *British Journal of Cancer*, 52:669–673.

Hardcastle JD. et al. (1996) Randomised controlled trial of faecal–occult–blood screening for colorectal cancer. *Lancet*, 348: 1472–1477.

Harvey BJ. et al. (1997) Effect of breast self–examination techniques on the risk of death from breast cancer. *Canadian Medical Association Journal*, 157:1205–1212.

Henschke CI et al. (1999) Early lung cancer action project: overall design and findings from baseline screening. *Lancet*, 354:99–105.

Hunter DJ et al. (1996) Cohort studies of fat intake and the risk of breast cancer – a pooled analysis. *New England Journal of Medicine*, 334:356–361.

International Agency for Research on Cancer (1986) *Tobacco Smoking*. Lyon, (IARC Monographs on the Carcinogenic Risk of Chemicals to Humans, Vol. 38).

International Agency for Research on Cancer (1988) *Alcohol Drinking*. Lyon, (IARC Monographs on the Evaluation of the Carcinogenic Risk of Chemicals to Humans, Vol. 44).

International Agency for Research on Cancer (1990) *Chromium, Nickel and Welding*. Lyon, (IARC Monographs on the Carcinogenic Risk of Chemicals to Humans, Vol. 49).

International Agency for Research on Cancer (1992) *Solar and Ultraviolet Radiation*. Lyon, (IARC Monographs on the Carcinogenic Risk of Chemicals to Humans, Vol. 55).

International Agency for Research on Cancer (1993) *Some Naturally Occurring Substances: Food Items and Constituents, Heterocyclic Aromatic Amines, and Mycotoxins*. Lyon, (IARC Monographs on the Carcinogenic Risk of Chemicals to Humans, Vol. 56).

International Agency for Research on Cancer (1994a) *Schistosomes, Liver Flukes and Helicobacter pylori*. Lyon, (IARC Monographs on the Carcinogenic Risk of Chemicals to Humans, Vol. 61).

International Agency for Research on Cancer (1994b) *Hepatitis Viruses*. Lyon, (IARC Monographs on the Carcinogenic Risk of Chemicals to Humans, Vol. 59).

International Agency for Research on Cancer (1995) *Human Papillomaviruses*. Lyon, (IARC Monographs on the Carcinogenic Risk of Chemicals to Humans, Vol. 64).

International Agency for Research on Cancer (1996) *Some Pharmaceutical Drugs*. Lyon, (IARC Monographs on the Evaluation of the Carcinogenic Risk of Chemicals to Humans, Vol. 66).

International Agency for Research on Cancer (1997) *Epstein–Barr virus and Kaposi's Sarcoma Herpesvirus/Human Herpesvirus 8* Lyon, (IARC Monographs on the Carcinogenic Risk of Chemicals to Humans, Vol. 70).

International Agency for Research on Cancer (1998a) *Carotenoids*. Lyon. (IARC Handbooks of cancer prevention Vol. 2).

International Agency for Research on Cancer (1998b) *Vitamin A*. Lyon. (IARC Handbooks of cancer prevention Vol. 3).

International Agency for Research on Cancer (1999) *Hormonal Contraception and Post–Menopausal Hormonal Therapy*. Lyon. (IARC Monographs on the Carcinogenic Risk of Chemicals to Humans, Vol. 72).

International Agency for Research on Cancer (2000) *Sunscreens*. Lyon. (IARC Handbooks of cancer prevention Vol. 5).

International Agency for Research on Cancer (2001) *Physical activity and weight reduction*. Lyon. (IARC Handbooks of cancer prevention Vol. 6).

International Agency for Research on Cancer (In press) *Breast Cancer Screening*. Lyon. IARC Handbooks of cancer prevention Vol. 7

International Organization for Standardization ISO, (2001) *ISO Standards Compendium: ISO 9000 – Quality Management Ed. 9*, Geneva, ISO

International Prostate Screening Trial Evaluation Group (1999) Rationale for randomised trials of prostate cancer screening. *European Journal of Cancer*, 35:262–271.

Jayant K et al. (1998) Survival from cervical cancer in Barshi registry, rural India. In: *Cancer survival in developing countries*. IARC Scientific Publication No. 145, pp: 69–77.

Jensen OM at al.,eds. (1991) *Cancer registration principles and methods*. Lyon, France: International Agency for Research on Cancer.

Joint WHO/FAO expert consultation on diet, nutrition and the prevention of chronic diseases, in preparation. WHO, Geneva.

Kato H, Schull WJ (1982) Studies of the mortality of A-bomb survivors. 7. Mortality, 1950–1978: Part I. Cancer mortality. *Radiation Research*, 90:395–432.

Key TJ, et al. (In preparation) Annex 5: The scientific basis for diet, nutrition and the prevention of cancer. In: *Diet, nutrition and the prevention of chronic diseases*. Joint WHO/FAO expert consultation on diet, nutrition and the prevention of chronic diseases. Geneva, WHO.

Kronborg O et al. (1996) Randomized study of screening for colorectal cancer with faecal-occult-blood test. *Lancet*, 348:1467–1471.

Lanier AP et al. (1973) Cancer and stilbestrol: a follow–up of 1719 persons exposed to estrogens in utero and born 1943–1959. *Mayo Clinic Proceedings*, 48:793–799.

Levin CV, El Gueddari B, Meghzifene A, (1999) Radiation therapy in Africa: distribution and equipment. *Radiotherapy and Oncology*, **52**: 79–84.

Liebeskind JC. (1991) Pain *can* kill. *Pain* 44: 3–4.

MacDonald N. (1991) Palliative care – the fourth phase of cancer prevention. In: *Cancer Detection and Prevention*. Boca Raton, Florida. Vol. 15, Issue 3, pp253–255. CRC Press Inc..

Mandel JS et al. (1993) Reducing mortality from colorectal cancer by screening for fecal occult blood. *New England Journal of medicine*, 328:1365–1371.

Mandel JS et al. (1999) Colorectal cancer mortality: Effectiveness of biennial screening for fecal occult blood. *Journal of the National Cancer Institute*, 91:434–437.

Mathew B et al., (1995) Evaluation of mouth self–examination in the control of oral cancer. *Br J Cancer* 71, 397–399.

Meredith C et al. (1996) Information needs of cancer patients in west Scotland: cross–sectional survey of patients' views. *British Medical Journal* 313: 724–6.

Mertens DM (1999) Inclusive evaluation: implications of transformative theory for evaluation. *South American Journal of Evaluation*, 20: 1–14.

Miller AB. (1984) The information explosion. The role of the epidemiologist. *Cancer Forum*, 8:67–75.

Miller AB. (1992) Cervical cancer screening programmes: managerial guidelines. Geneva, World Health Organization.

Miller AB. (1999) Tobacco and cancer: what has been, and could be, achieved? *Cancer Strategy*, 1:165–169.

Miller AB et al. (1989) Mortality from breast cancer after radiation during fluoroscopic examination in patients being treated for tuberculosis. *New England Journal of Medicine*, 321:1285–1289.

Miller AB et al. (1990) Report of a workshop of the UICC project on evaluation of screening for cancer. *International Journal of Cancer*, 46:761–769.

Miller AB et al. (2000a) Canadian National Breast Screening Study–2: 13–year results of a randomized trial in women age 50–59 years. *Journal of the National Cancer Institute*, 92:1490–1499.

Miller AB et al. (2000b) Report on consensus conference on cervical cancer screening and management. *International Journal of Cancer*, 86:440–447.

National Cancer Institute (U.S.) (2002) *The nation's investment in cancer research:a budget proposal for fiscal year 2003.* Prepared by the Director, National Cancer Institute, National Institute of Health. Bethesda, The National Cancer Institute.

Newcomb PA et al. (1992) Screening sigmoidoscopy and colorectal cancer mortality. *Journal of the National Cancer Institute*, 84:1572–1575.

Omenn GS et al. (1996) Effects of a combination of beta carotene and vitamin A on lung cancer and cardiovascular disease. *New England Journal of Medicine*, 334: 1150–1155.

Parkin DM et al Ed. (1997) *Cancer Incidence in Five Continents*, Vol. VII. Lyon, International Agency for Research on Cancer, 1997 (IARC Scientific Publications, No. 143).

Peto R et al. (1994) *Mortality from smoking in developed countries, 1950–2000*. New York, Oxford University Press.

Pisani P, Parkin DM, Munoz N, Ferlay J (1997) Cancer and infection: estimates of the attributable fraction in 1990. *Cancer Epidemiology Biomarkers and Prevention* 6:387–400.

Ponten J et al. (1995) Strategies for control of cervical cancer. *International Journal of Cancer*, 60:1– 26.

Prorok PC et al. (1984) UICC workshop on evaluation of screening programmes for cancer. *International Journal of Cancer*, 34:1–4.

Rankin JG, Ashley MJ. (1985) Alcohol–related health problems and their prevention. In: Last J, ed. *Public health and preventive medicine*, 12th ed. Norwalk, CT, Appleton–Century–Crofts, 1039–1073.

Salas I. (2001) Methodology for the reorganization of the cervical cancer programme in Chile. World Health Organization Technical Document WHO/PCC/122E/2001 (unpublished).

Sankaranarayanan R et al. (1997) Visual inspection as a screening test for cervical cancer control in developing countries. In: Fanco E, Monsonego J eds. *New developments in cervical cancer screening and prevention*. Oxford, Blackwell Science, pp: 411–421.

Sankaranarayanan R, Black RJ, Parkin DM. ed.s (1998) *Cancer Survival in Developing Countries*. Lyon.. IARC Scientific Publications no 145.

Sankaranarayanan R et al. (2000) Early findings from a community based cluster randomised oral cancer screening intervention trial in Kerala, India. *Cancer* 88:664–773.

Sasieni PD, Cuzick J, Lynch FE. (1996) Estimating the efficacy of screening by auditing smear histories of women with and without cervical cancer. The National Coordinating Network for Cervical Screening Working Group. *British Journal of Cancer*, 73:1001–1005.

Selby J et al. (1992) A case–control study of screening sigmoidoscopy and mortality from colorectal cancer. *New England Journal of Medicine*, 326:653–657.

Sell L et al. (1993) Communicating the diagnosis of lung cancer. *Respiratory Medicine* 87:61–3.

Shapiro S. (1997) Periodic screening for breast cancer: The HIP randomized controlled trial. *Monographs, Journal of the National Cancer Institute*, 22:27–30.

Sikora K et al. (1999) Essential drugs for cancer therapy. *Annals of Oncology*, 10:385–390.

Simpson M et al. (1991) Doctor–patient communication: the Toronto consensus statement. *British Medical Journal* 303:1385–7.

Stanley K. (1993) Control of tobacco production and use. In: Jamison D, et al. eds. *Disease control priorities in developing countries*. New York, Oxford University Press, pp: 703–723.

Stjernswärd J. (1985) Cancer control: strategies and priorities. *World Health Forum*, 6:160–164.

Stjernswärd J. (1993) Palliative medicine – a global perspective. In: Doyle D et al. eds *Oxford Textbook of Palliative Medicine*. Oxford, Oxford University Press. 803–816.

The Alpha–Tocopherol, Beta Carotene Cancer Prevention Study Group (1994). The effect of vitamin E and beta carotene on the incidence of lung cancer and other cancers in male smokers. *New England Journal of Medicine*, 330: 1029–1035.

Tisdale M. (1997) Cancer cachexia. *Journal of the National Cancer Institute* 89:1763–1773.

Tomatis L et al., eds. (1990) *Cancer: Causes, Occurrence and Control.* Lyon. International Agency for Research on Cancer, (IARC Scientific Publication, No. 100).

Tubiana M, (1999) Cancer Prevention. *Acta Oncologica,* 38: 689–694.

Twycross R. (1994) *Pain relief in advanced cancer.* Edinburgh. Churchill Livingstone.

Ullrich A, Fitzgerald P. (1990) Stress experienced by physicians and nurses in the cancer ward. *Social Science and Medicine,* 31:1013–1022.

United Nations Development Programme (1998) Capacity assessment and development, Technical Advisory Paper No. 3 Management Development and Governance Division.

US Department of Health, Education, and Welfare. (1964) *Smoking and health. A report of the advisory committee to the Surgeon–General of the Public Health Service.* U.S. Department of Health, Education, and Welfare, Public Health Service, Communicable Disease Center DHJEW Publication No. 1103.

US Department of Health and Human Services (1984) Clinical Practice Guideline Number 9. *Management of cancer pain.* Public Health Service, Agency for Health Care Policy and Research. AHCPR Publication No. 94–0592: 8.

Vineis P et al. (1988) Proportion of lung cancers in males due to occupation in different areas of the U.S. *International Journal of Cancer,* 42: 851–856.

Weiss CH (1998) *Evaluation.* Englwood Cliffs NJ, Prentice–Hall.

World Cancer Research Fund & American Institute for Cancer Research (1997). *Food, Nutrition and the Prevention of Cancer: A Global Perspective.* Washington, DC, American Institute for Cancer Research.

World Health Organization (1963) *Annual Epidemiological and Vital Statistics 1960.* Geneva, WHO.

World Health Organization (1981) *World Health Statistics Annual 1980–81.* Geneva, WHO.

World Health Organization (1984) Control of oral cancer in developing countries. *Bulletin of the World Health Organization,* 62:817–830.

World Health Organization (1986a). The use of quantitative methods in planning national cancer control programmes. *Bulletin of the World Health Organization,* 64:683–693.

World Health Organization (1986b) Control of cancer of the cervix uteri. *Bulletin of the World Health Organization,* 1986, 64:607–618.

World Health Organization (1986c) *Ottawa Charter for Health Promotion.* An international conference on health promotion the move towards a new public health, Nov 17–21 1986 Ottawa.

World Health Organization (1990a) *Diet, nutrition and the prevention of chronic disease. Report of a WHO Study Group.* Geneva, (WHO Technical Report Series, No. 797).

World Health Organization (1990b) Cancer pain relief and palliative care. Report of a WHO Expert Committee, WHO, Geneva.

World Health Organization (1992) The international statistical classification of diseases and related health problems, tenth revision. WHO, Geneva, Vol. 1

World Health Organization (1996). Cancer pain relief: with a guide to opioid availability. 2nd edition. WHO, Geneva.

World Health Organization (1998a). *Cancer pain relief and palliative care in children.* WHO, Geneva.

World Health Organization (1998b). *Symptom relief in terminal illness.* WHO, Geneva.

World Health Organization (1998c) *Guidelines for the controlling and monitoring the tobacco epidemic.* Geneva, WHO.

World Health Organization (2001a) *Cervical cancer screening in developing countries.* Report of a WHO consultation 27–30 March 2001.

World Health Organization (2001b) *Assessment of national capacity for noncommunicable disease prevention and control. The report of a global survey.* Geneva, WHO.

World Health Organization (2001c) The World Health Report 2001 Mental Health: New understanding, new hope. Geneva, WHO.

Wulsin LR. (2000) Does Depression Kill? *Archives of Internal Medicine,* 160: 1731–1732.

Yach D. (2001) Chronic disease and disability of the poor: tackling the challenge. *Development,* 44: 59–65.